HYPOTHYROIDISM COOKBOOK

"The Ultimate Guide To Easy, Quick, And Healthy Recipes To Combat The Unsuspected Illness And Support Women's Thyroid Health And Weight Loss."

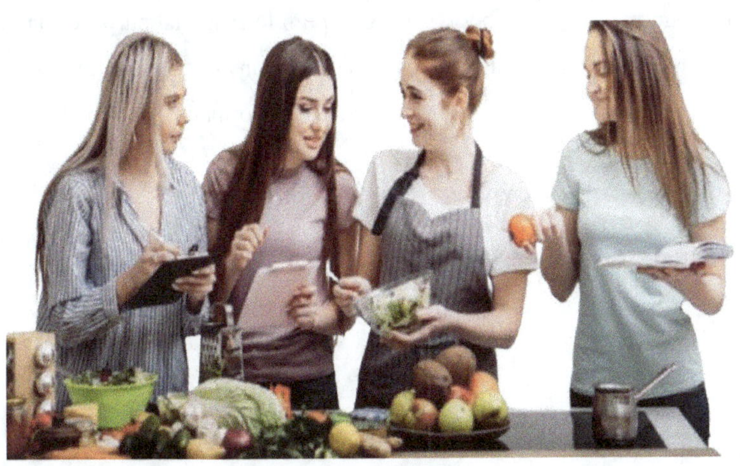

AVELINE WINTER

TABLE OF CONTENT

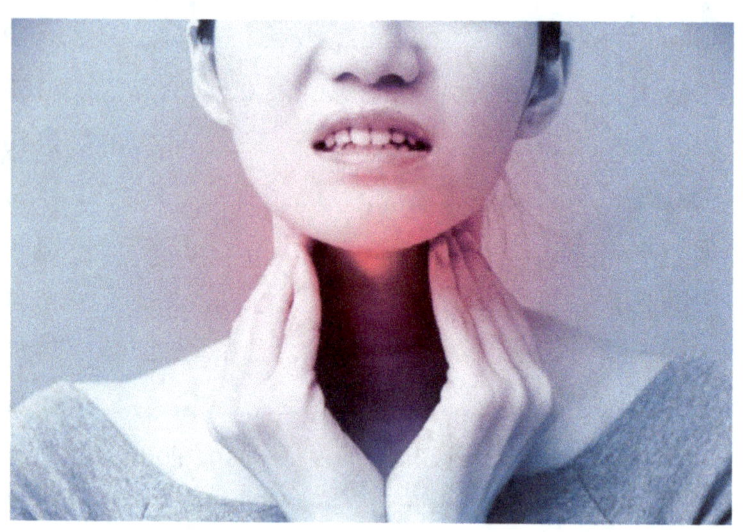

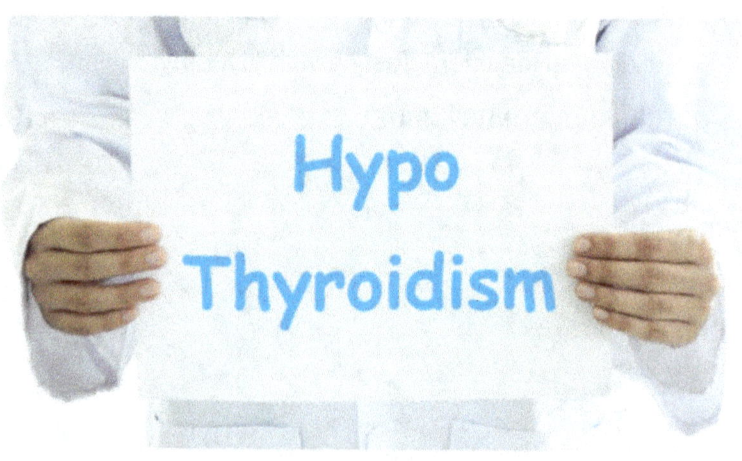

Hypo
Thyroidism

INTRODUCTION

As a cookbook writer and nutritionist, I have seen firsthand the transformative power of food in managing hypothyroidism. When my mother was diagnosed with this condition when I was young, she struggled to find foods that she could eat and enjoy. Watching her go through this experience inspired me to become a professional nutritionist and chef, dedicated to creating delicious and nutritious meals that support individuals with hypothyroidism.

That's why I am thrilled to introduce you to the Hypothyroidism Cookbook, a collection of quick, easy, and healthy recipes designed to provide quick relief and support for a healthier thyroid and a longer life. This cookbook is a comprehensive guide to using food as medicine, offering an essential introduction that explains the thyroid-diet connection and provides instruction on foods to eat and avoid, along with guidelines for preparing your meals.

The Hypothyroidism Cookbook is a valuable resource for anyone looking to manage their hypothyroidism through diet. It offers a variety of recipes that are not only delicious but also nutrient-dense, providing essential nutrients such as iodine, selenium, and zinc that can help maintain a healthy thyroid function. The cookbook also includes allergy-friendly options and ingredient substitutions, making it accessible to individuals with specific dietary restrictions.

One of the unique features of this cookbook is its emphasis on quick and easy recipes that can be prepared in just 30 minutes. This makes it an ideal resource for busy individuals who want to eat healthily but don't have a lot of time to spend in the kitchen.

The Hypothyroidism Cookbook is also a great resource for those who want to learn more about the science behind hypothyroidism and how food can be used to manage this condition.

The Hypothyroidism Cookbook is a must-have resource for anyone looking to manage their hypothyroidism through diet. It offers a wealth of information, delicious recipes, and practical tips that can help you take control of your health and well-being. Don't miss out on the opportunity to discover the power of food in managing hypothyroidism.

- Understanding Hypothyroidism

Explaining the Condition and its Impact on Diet Hypothyroidism is a common condition in which the thyroid gland does not produce enough thyroid hormone, leading to various symptoms and potential impacts on diet. The thyroid is a small gland at the front of the neck that produces hormones regulating the body's metabolism. More than 12 percent of the U.S. population will experience a thyroid condition at some point in their lives, with one in eight women developing a thyroid disorder during their lifetime.

Hypothyroidism, also known as an underactive thyroid, can result from an autoimmune disorder such as Hashimoto's disease, where the immune system attacks the thyroid gland. This can lead to fatigue, unexplained weight gain, depression, constipation, and other symptoms. It is essential to highlight the importance of timely evaluation for this condition.

Impact on Diet

Hypothyroidism can impact diet and weight. Due to the slowed metabolism associated with hypothyroidism, individuals may experience weight gain or have difficulty losing weight. In some cases, there may be a need for dietary adjustments, such as ensuring an adequate intake of iodine and selenium, which are essential for thyroid function. Additionally, some individuals with hypothyroidism may benefit from a well-balanced diet that supports overall health and helps manage symptoms, such as fatigue and constipation.

By understanding hypothyroidism and its potential impact on diet, individuals can make informed decisions and seek the necessary support to manage the condition effectively.

- Nutrition and Its Role in Managing Hypothyroidism

Like we discussed earlier, hypothyroidism is a condition in which the thyroid gland does not produce enough thyroid hormone, leading to various symptoms and potential impacts on diet. Nutrition plays a crucial role in managing hypothyroidism, and a well-balanced diet can help improve thyroid function and symptoms.

Nutrients Critical for Thyroid Function

Several nutrients are critical for thyroid function, including iodine, selenium, iron, zinc, and vitamins B12, D3, and A. Iodine is essential for the thyroid to work as it should, and getting enough iodine in the diet is crucial. Selenium is also important for thyroid function, as it helps convert thyroid hormones into their active form. Iron and zinc are necessary for the production of thyroid hormones, and vitamin B12 is essential for the metabolism of thyroid hormones. Vitamin D3 is also important for thyroid function, as it helps regulate the immune system and reduce inflammation. Vitamin A is necessary for the production of thyroid hormones and helps regulate the thyroid gland.

Foods to Eat and Avoid

A diet rich in whole, nutrient-dense foods like vegetables, fruits, nuts, and whole grains is beneficial for individuals with hypothyroidism. It is also important to limit pro-inflammatory foods with added sugar or ultra-processed foods. Additionally, some individuals with hypothyroidism may benefit from a well-balanced diet that supports overall health and helps manage symptoms, such as fatigue and constipation.

It is recommended to avoid excessive amounts of iodine, either in medications or supplements, as this could potentially alter your thyroid hormone level. It is also important to limit foods high in soy protein, as large amounts of soy might interfere with the absorption of thyroid hormone.

Mediterranean Diet

The Mediterranean diet is increasingly being prescribed for individuals with hypothyroidism, especially those suffering from Hashimoto's thyroiditis. This diet is rich in critical elements, including iodine, selenium, iron, zinc, and vitamins B12, D3, and A. It is also high in antioxidants, building up an anti-inflammatory profile, reducing thyroid autoantibodies and body fat, and improving thyroid function.

Nutrition plays a crucial role in managing hypothyroidism, and a well-balanced diet rich in whole, nutrient-dense foods can help improve thyroid function and symptoms.

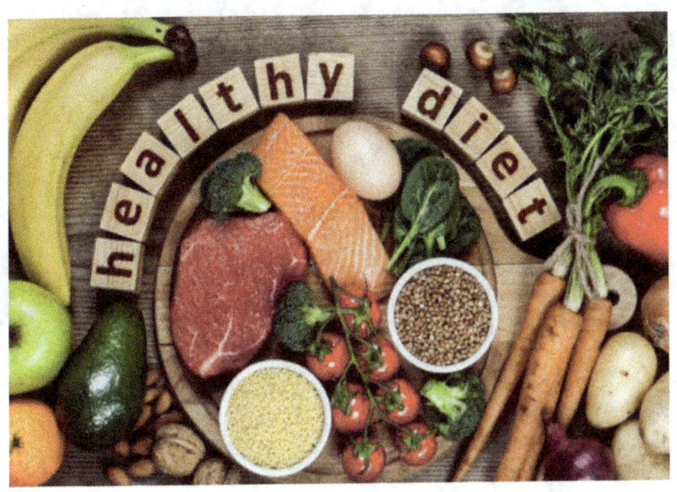

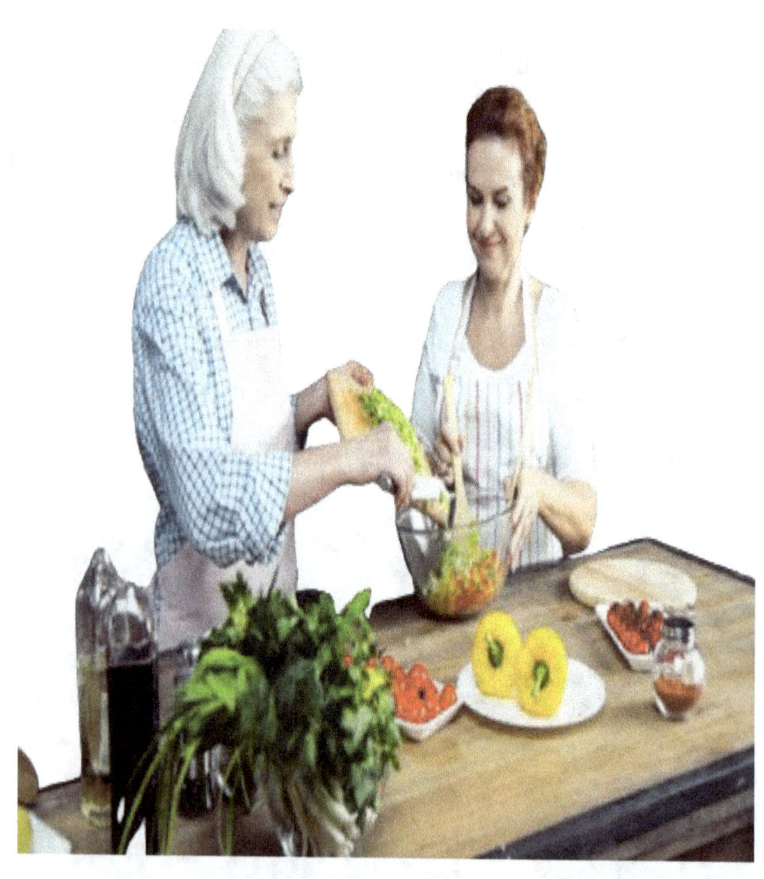

CHAPTER 1

Energizing Breakfasts

Are you ready to learn about hypothyroidism and how to make some delicious breakfasts that will help you manage your condition? Well, you've come to the right place!

First things first, let's talk about why breakfast is so important for those with hypothyroidism. A nutritious breakfast can help kickstart your metabolism and provide the energy you need to tackle the day. Plus, getting enough iodine in your diet is essential for your thyroid to function properly, and breakfast is a great opportunity to get some of those essential nutrients in.

Now, I know what you're thinking - "healthy breakfasts are boring and tasteless." But fear not, my friend! Chapter 1 of this book is all about "Energizing Breakfasts," and we've got some delicious recipes that will make your taste buds dance with joy. We're talking about whole, nutrient-dense foods like fruits, vegetables, and whole grains that will not only support your thyroid function but also taste amazing.

So, are you ready to start your day off right with some delicious and nutritious breakfasts? Let's do this!

- Sunrise Smoothie Bowl

Overview:

This vibrant and nutritious sunrise smoothie bowl is specifically tailored to support individuals with hypothyroidism. Packed with thyroid-friendly ingredients, this delicious meal is designed to help balance thyroid function, reduce stress, fatigue, weight gain, and alleviate symptoms.

Ingredients:

- 1 frozen banana
- 1/2 cup frozen mango
- 1/2 cup frozen pineapple
- 1/2 cup spinach
- 1/2 cup unsweetened almond milk
- 1 tablespoon chia seeds
- 1 tablespoon ground flaxseed
- 1/2 teaspoon grated fresh ginger

- Toppings: sliced strawberries, blueberries, and unsweetened coconut flakes

Step-by-Step Instructions:

1. In a blender, combine the frozen banana, frozen mango, frozen pineapple, spinach, almond milk, chia seeds, ground flaxseed, and grated ginger.

2. Blend until it is smooth and creamy, adding more almond milk if needed to reach the desired consistency.

3. Pour the smoothie into a bowl and top with sliced strawberries, blueberries, and unsweetened coconut flakes.

Nutritional Information:

- Calories: Approximately 350

- Protein: 7g

- Fat: 10g

- Carbohydrates: 60g

- Fiber: 12g

Variations/Ingredient Substitutions:

- For a nut-free option, substitute the almond milk with coconut milk or oat milk.

- Replace the spinach with kale for an extra boost of nutrients.

- Add a scoop of high-quality protein powder to increase the protein content.

Serving Tip:

Enjoy the sunrise smoothie bowl as a refreshing and nourishing breakfast or snack. Serve it cold for a refreshing start to your day.

Bonus Health Tip:

Incorporate selenium-rich foods such as Brazil nuts, zinc-rich foods like pumpkin seeds, and iodine-rich ingredients such as seaweed to further support thyroid health. Additionally, maintaining a well-balanced diet with adequate levels of vitamins and minerals is essential for individuals with hypothyroidism.

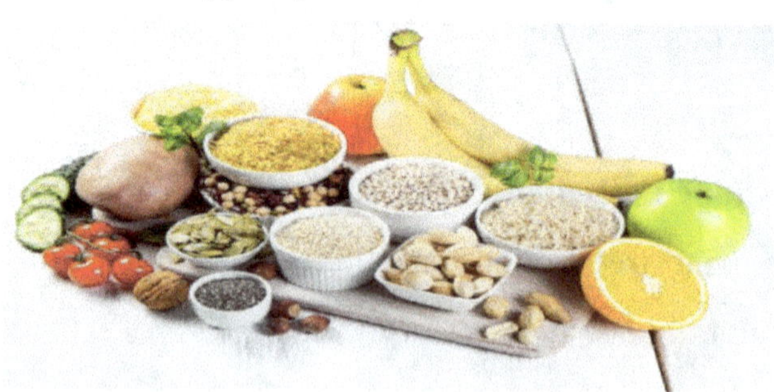

- Quinoa Power Porridge

Get ready to power up your morning with a delicious and nutritious bowl of Quinoa Power Porridge. This superfood-packed porridge is not only easy to make and tasty but also comes with benefits that can help in managing hypothyroidism. Quinoa is a gluten-free superfood that contains all nine essential amino acids, making it a complete source of protein, which is beneficial for those with hypothyroidism, as protein is important for thyroid function. The recipe is versatile and can be tailored to meet various dietary needs, including gluten-free, dairy-free, vegan, and vegetarian. Now, let's dive into the details.

Ingredients

- 1 cup quinoa
- 1 cup oats
- 2 cups almond milk
- 1 cup water
- 1 teaspoon cinnamon
- 2 tablespoons maple syrup or honey
- 2 tablespoons hemp seeds
- 2 tablespoons chia seeds

- 2 tablespoons flaxseed meal

- Toppings of your choice: fresh berries, sliced fruit, nuts, seeds, and nut butter

Step-by-Step Instructions

1. In a small pot, combine the quinoa, oats, almond milk, water, and cinnamon. Bring the liquid to a boil.

2. Remove the porridge from the heat and stir in the maple syrup or honey, hemp seeds, chia seeds, and flaxseed meal.

3. Divide the porridge equally between two bowls and top with your favorite toppings, such as fresh berries, sliced fruit, nuts, seeds, and a drizzle of nut butter.

Nutritional Information

The nutritional content may vary based on the specific ingredients and toppings used. However, quinoa is a good source of protein, fiber, and various vitamins and minerals, which are beneficial for individuals with hypothyroidism.

Dietary Variations

- Gluten-Free: Ensure that all ingredients, including oats, are certified gluten-free.

- Dairy-Free: Use dairy-free milk, such as almond milk or coconut milk.
- Vegan/Vegetarian: This recipe is already vegan. Ensure that the toppings and sweeteners are vegan-friendly.
- Keto/Pescetarian: Adjust the toppings and sweeteners to align with the keto or pescetarian diet.

Serving Tip

For an extra indulgent touch, drizzle the porridge with a bit of almond or peanut butter and top it with your favorite fruits, nuts, and seeds.

Bonus Health Tip

Consider adding a source of iodine to the porridge, such as iodized salt or seaweed, as iodine is essential for thyroid health.

This Quinoa Power Porridge is a fantastic way to start your day, especially if you're looking to support your hypothyroidism management. Enjoy your nutritious and delicious breakfast!

- Avocado Toast Variations

Are you looking for a delicious and healthy recipe that can help heal hypothyroidism? Look no further than Avocado Toast Variations! Avocado is a superfood that is rich in healthy fats, fiber, and other nutrients that can help decrease inflammation and support optimal thyroid hormones. This recipe is easy to make and can be customized to meet different dietary needs, such as gluten-free, dairy-free, lactose-free, vegan, vegetarian, keto, and pescetarian. Here are the ingredients and step-by-step instructions:

Ingredients:

- 2 slices of bread (gluten-free optional)

- 1 ripe avocado

- 1/4 teaspoon of sea salt

- 1/4 teaspoon of black pepper

- Optional toppings: sliced tomatoes, microgreens, smoked salmon, boiled eggs, or hummus

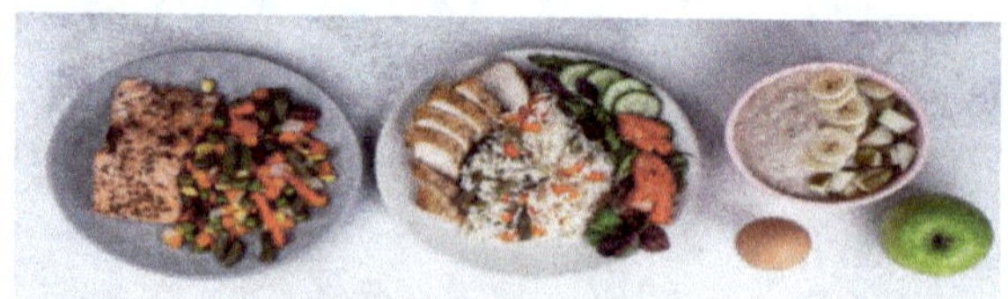

Instructions:

1. Toast the bread slices until golden brown.

2. Cut the avocado in half, remove the pit, and scoop out the flesh into a bowl.

3. Mash the avocado with a fork and add sea salt and black pepper to taste.

4. Spread the avocado mixture evenly on the toast slices.

5. Add your desired toppings, such as sliced tomatoes, microgreens, smoked salmon, boiled eggs, or hummus.

6. Serve and enjoy!

Nutritional Information:

- Calories: 250
- Total Fat: 15g
- Saturated Fat: 2g
- Cholesterol: 0mg
- Sodium: 300mg
- Total Carbohydrates: 25g
- Dietary Fiber: 10g
- Sugars: 2g
- Protein: 6g

It is important to avoid certain foods that can interfere with thyroid function, such as soy, gluten, and processed foods. This recipe is gluten-free and can be made dairy-free and vegan by using gluten-free bread and skipping the optional toppings that contain dairy or animal products. For a keto-friendly version, use keto bread and skip the toppings that contain carbs. For a pescetarian version, add smoked salmon as a topping.

Serving Tip:

Avocado Toast Variations can be served as a healthy breakfast, lunch, or snack. It is a great way to start your day with a nutrient-dense and satisfying meal that can keep you full and energized for hours.

Bonus Health Tip:

In addition to eating a healthy diet, it is important to manage stress, exercise regularly, and get enough sleep to support optimal thyroid function. Incorporate stress-relieving hobbies such as yoga, meditation, or deep breathing techniques into your daily routine. Most days of the week, aim for at least 30 minutes of moderate-intensity activity, such as brisk walking or cycling. And make sure to get 7-9 hours of sleep each night to support optimal hormonal balance.

- Nutrient-Rich Breakfast Muffins

Are you ready to kick-start your day with a delicious and nutritious breakfast that can support your thyroid health? These nutrient-rich breakfast muffins are not only a tasty treat but also packed with ingredients that can help heal hypothyroidism. The recipe is versatile and can be customized to meet various dietary needs, including gluten-free, dairy-free, and vegetarian options. Let's dive into the details!

Benefits:

Eggs, a key ingredient in the muffins, are a great source of protein, which is essential for supporting thyroid function. Additionally, the use of ingredients like banana, peanut butter, and oats provides a good balance of complex carbohydrates, healthy fats, and fiber, which can help stabilize blood sugar levels and support energy production, both of which are beneficial for individuals with hypothyroidism.

Ingredients:

- 1 large mashed banana

- 1/3 cup natural peanut butter

- 1 large egg

- 3/4 cup rolled oats

- 1/2 teaspoon pure vanilla extract

- 1/2 teaspoon baking powder

- Optional mix-ins: nuts, berries, chocolate chips

Instructions:

1. Preheat the oven to 375°F.

2. In a bowl, mash the ripe banana and then add the egg, natural peanut butter, and pure vanilla extract. Mix well.

3. Stir in the rolled oats and baking powder until all ingredients are well combined.

4. If desired, add your choice of mix-ins, such as nuts, berries, or chocolate chips.

5. Pour the batter into a muffin tin lined with parchment paper, filling each cup about 3/4 full.

6. Bake for 22-25 minutes or until the muffins are light and golden.

7. Enjoy the muffins warm, with a spread of salted butter or your favorite topping.

Nutritional Information:

- Serving Size: 1 muffin

- Calories: Approximately 200

- Total Fat: 10-12g

- Carbohydrates: 20-25g

- Protein: 6-8g

- Fiber: 3-4g

Variations:

- For a gluten-free version, use certified gluten-free oats.

- To make the muffins dairy-free, ensure the peanut butter used is free from added dairy ingredients.

- Vegetarians can enjoy these muffins as is, while those following a pescetarian diet may consider adding inclusions like omega-3 rich walnuts.

Serving Tip:

These nutrient-rich breakfast muffins are perfect for a quick and satisfying breakfast. They can also be enjoyed as a convenient on-the-go snack to help maintain energy levels throughout the day.

Bonus Health Tip:

In addition to enjoying these delicious muffins, consider pairing them with a source of clean protein, such as a side of Greek yogurt or a boiled egg, to create a well-rounded breakfast that can further support your thyroid health.

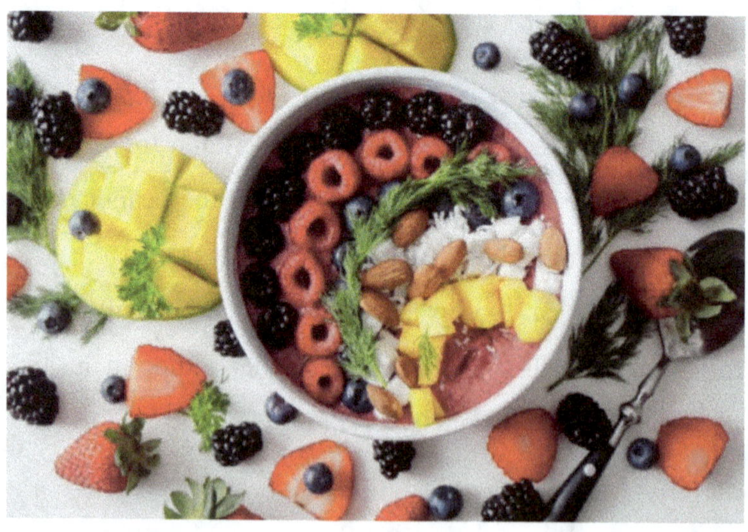

CHAPTER 2

Nourishing Soups and Salads

In Chapter 2 of our exploration into hypothyroidism, we delve into the realm of nourishing soups and salads. Hypothyroidism, characterized by low levels of thyroid hormone, can have diverse manifestations and impacts on health if left untreated. This common condition can be caused by various factors, such as autoimmune thyroid disease or lack of iodine in the diet. The clinical presentation of hypothyroidism varies, and its diagnosis is easily made through simple blood tests. Through the lens of this chapter, we will uncover the significance of wholesome soups and salads in supporting individuals with hypothyroidism, offering insights into nutrient-rich ingredients and delicious recipes to aid in managing this condition. Join us on this journey of culinary exploration, where we will discover the vital role of nourishing foods in the context of hypothyroidism.

- Thyroid-Boosting Green Salad

This salad is packed with nutrient-dense ingredients that can help support optimal thyroid health. The recipe is vegan and can be customized to meet various dietary needs, including gluten-free and dairy-free options. Let's dive into the details!

Benefits for Hypothyroidism:

This salad is rich in greens, which are a great source of vitamins and minerals that can support thyroid function. The use of ingredients like tomatoes, celery, and chia seeds provides a good balance of antioxidants, fiber, and healthy fats, which can help decrease inflammation and support energy production, both of which are beneficial for individuals with hypothyroidism.

Ingredients:

- 3 cups of chopped green lettuce or microgreens

- 3 medium tomatoes

- 1 medium stalk of celery

- 1 spring onion

- 1 tablespoon chia seeds

- 1 tablespoon pumpkin seeds

- 2 Brazil nuts

Instructions:

1. Wash the lettuce or microgreens and chop them into small pieces.

2. Place the chopped salad leaves into a bowl.

3. Wash the tomatoes, celery, and spring onion and chop them into pieces.

4. Blend together the tomatoes, celery, and spring onion along with the chia seeds, pumpkin seeds, and Brazil nuts.

5. Pour the blended sauce over the salad leaves and mix well.

6. Serve and enjoy!

Variations:

- For a gluten-free version, ensure all ingredients are gluten-free.

- To make the salad dairy-free, skip any optional toppings that contain dairy.

- Vegetarians and vegans can enjoy this salad as is.

Nutritional Information:

- Serving Size: 1 salad

- Calories: Approximately 200

- Total Fat: 10-12g

- Carbohydrates: 20-25g

- Protein: 6-8g

- Fiber: 3-4g

Serving Tip:

This Thyroid-Boosting Green Salad is perfect for a light and refreshing lunch or dinner. It can be served as a side dish or as a main course by adding a source of protein, such as grilled chicken or tofu.

Bonus Health Tip:

In addition to eating a healthy diet, it is important to manage stress, exercise regularly, and get enough sleep to support optimal thyroid function. Incorporate stress-relieving hobbies such as yoga, meditation, or deep breathing techniques into your daily routine. Most days of the week, aim for at least 30 minutes of moderate-intensity activity, such as brisk walking or cycling. And make sure to get 7-9 hours of sleep each night to support optimal hormonal balance.

- Roasted Vegetable Soup

This soup is packed with nutrient-dense ingredients that can help decrease inflammation and support optimal thyroid function. The recipe is vegan and can be customized to meet various dietary needs, including gluten-free and dairy-free options. Let's dive into the details!

Benefits for Hypothyroidism:

This soup is rich in roasted vegetables, which are a great source of vitamins and minerals that can support thyroid function. The use of ingredients like sweet potato, bell peppers, and garlic provides a good balance of antioxidants, fiber, and healthy fats, which can help decrease inflammation and support energy production, both of which are beneficial for individuals with hypothyroidism.

Ingredients:

- 1 red bell pepper, diced
- 1 medium peeled and diced sweet potato (about 1 pound)
- 1 yellow squash or zucchini, diced
- 1 small head of cauliflower, diced
- 1 medium white onion, diced

- 2 tablespoons olive oil, divided

- Fine sea salt and freshly-cracked black pepper

- 4 cloves garlic, minced

- 2 to 3 cups vegetable broth

- Optional toppings: fresh thyme, grated Parmesan cheese (or vegan alternative)

Instructions:

1. Preheat the oven to 400°F.

2. In a large bowl, toss the diced vegetables with 1 tablespoon of olive oil, sea salt, and black pepper.

3. Spread the vegetables in a single layer on a baking sheet and roast for 20-25 minutes or until tender and lightly browned.

4. In a large pot, heat the remaining olive oil over medium-high heat.

5. Add the minced garlic and sauté for 1-2 minutes, stirring occasionally, until fragrant.

6. Add the roasted vegetables and vegetable broth to the pot and stir to combine.

7. Bring the mixture to a boil, then reduce the heat and simmer for 10-15 minutes.

8. Use an immersion blender to puree the soup until smooth.

9. Season the soup with additional salt and pepper to taste.

10. Serve the soup warm, topped with fresh thyme and grated Parmesan cheese (or vegan alternative) if desired.

Variations:

- For a gluten-free version, ensure all ingredients are gluten-free.

- To make the soup dairy-free, skip the Parmesan cheese topping or use a vegan alternative.

- Vegetarians and vegans can enjoy this soup as is.

Nutritional Information:

- Serving Size: 1 cup

- Calories: Approximately 100

- Total Fat: 5-6g

- Carbohydrates: 12-15g

- Protein: 2-3g

- Fiber: 3-4g

Serving Tip:

This Roasted Vegetable Soup is perfect for a cozy and comforting meal. It can be served as a starter or as a main course by adding a side of crusty bread or a protein source, such as grilled chicken or tofu.

Bonus Health Tip:

In addition to eating a healthy diet, it is important to manage stress, exercise regularly, and get enough sleep to support optimal thyroid function. Incorporate stress-relieving hobbies such as yoga, meditation, or deep breathing techniques into your daily routine. Most days of the week, aim for at least 30 minutes of moderate-intensity activity, such as brisk walking or cycling. And make sure to get 7-9 hours of sleep each night to support optimal hormonal balance.

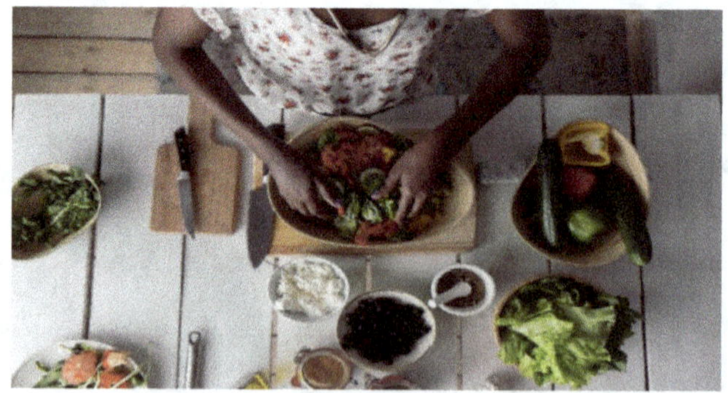

- Seaweed and Tofu Miso Soup

This soup is packed with ingredients that are beneficial for thyroid function, including wakame seaweed, which is rich in iodine, and miso paste, which is a fermented food that is rich in probiotics. The recipe is simple and easy to follow, and can be adapted to meet different dietary needs, such as gluten-free, dairy-free, vegan, or vegetarian. Here's how to make it:

Ingredients:

- 4 cups vegetable broth
- 1/2 cup of chopped green chard or another sturdy green
- 1/2 cup green onion, chopped
- 1/4 cup firm tofu, cubed
- 3-4 Tbsp white miso paste (fermented soybean paste)
- 1 sheet dried wakame, cut into large rectangles or small pieces
- 2 pinches kelp flakes

Instructions:

1. Place vegetable broth in a medium-sized saucepan and bring to a low simmer.

2. Add wakame and simmer for 5-7 minutes.

3. In the meantime, place miso (starting with the lesser end of the range) into a small bowl, add a little hot water and whisk until smooth.

4. Add chopped greens and tofu to the pot and cook for 5 minutes.

5. Remove from heat, then add miso mixture, and stir to combine.

6. Taste and add more miso, kelp flakes, or a pinch of pink salt if desired.

7. Serve warm.

Nutritional Information:

This recipe makes 4 servings. Each serving contains approximately:

- 80 calories

- 3g fat

- 8g carbohydrates

- 6g protein

- 2g fiber

Variations:

- Gluten-free: Use gluten-free miso paste and tamari instead of soy sauce.

- Dairy-free: Use a dairy-free vegetable broth and omit the tofu.

- Vegan: Follow the dairy-free variation and use a vegan miso paste.

- Vegetarian: Follow the vegan variation and add the tofu back in.

- Keto: Omit the green chard and use a low-carb vegetable broth.

- Pescetarian: Add cooked shrimp or fish to the soup.

- Lactose-free: Use a lactose-free vegetable broth.

Serving Tip:

Garnish with diced scallions and serve with a side of brown rice or quinoa for a complete meal.

Bonus Health Tip:

Seaweed is a great source of iodine, which is important for thyroid function. Incorporating seaweed into your diet can help prevent hypothyroidism and goiter. Try adding roasted wakame to your salads or snacking on nori seaweed chips for a healthy and delicious treat.

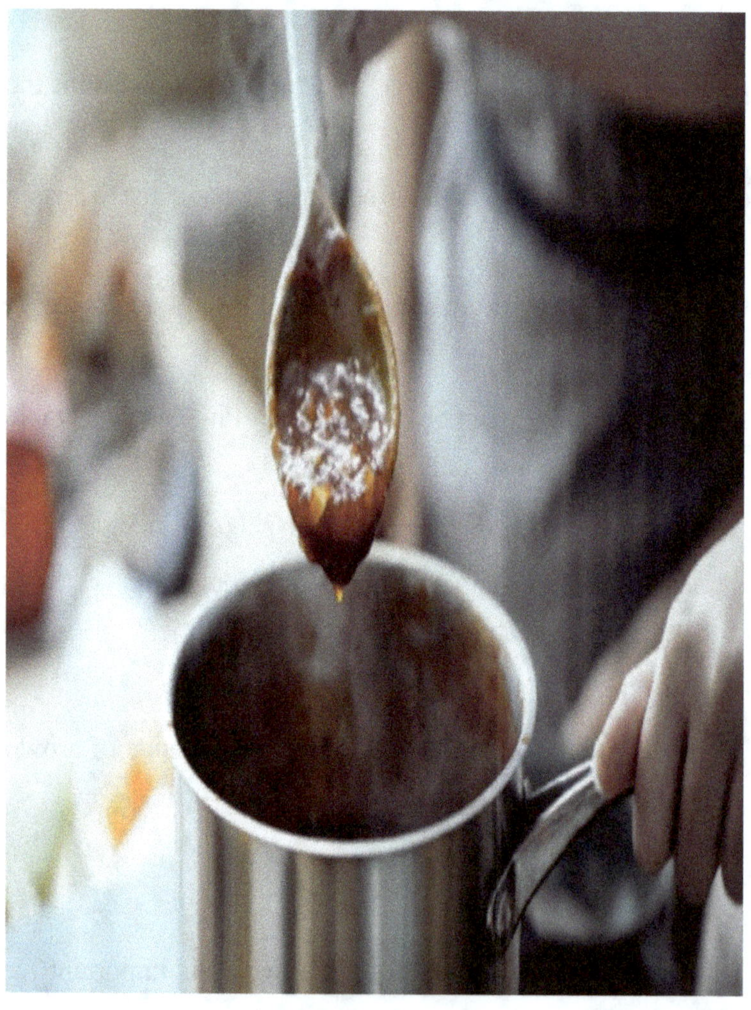

- Spinach and Lentil Salad

This salad is packed with ingredients that are beneficial for thyroid function, including spinach, which is rich in vitamins and minerals, and lentils, which are a great source of protein and fiber. The recipe is simple and easy to follow, and can be adapted to meet different dietary needs. Here's how to make it:

Ingredients:
- 1 pound spinach, washed and chopped
- 1 cup dry uncooked lentils
- 1 small onion, chopped
- 1 carrot, chopped
- 1 clove garlic, minced
- 1 bay leaf
- 1/3 cup pecans, chopped
- 1/4 cup olive oil
- 2 tbsp balsamic vinegar
- 1 tsp Dijon mustard
- Salt and pepper, to taste

Instructions:

1. In a medium pot, combine the lentils, onion, carrot, garlic, and bay leaf. Add enough water to cover the ingredients and bring to a boil.

2. Reduce heat and simmer for about 30 minutes, or until the lentils are tender.

3. Drain the lentils and discard the bay leaf, onion, and carrot.

4. In a large bowl, combine the chopped spinach and pecans.

5. In a separate small bowl, whisk together the olive oil, balsamic vinegar, and Dijon mustard to create a dressing.

6. Pour the dressing over the spinach and pecans, and toss to combine.

7. Add the cooked lentils to the salad and season with salt and pepper to taste.

8. Serve immediately.

Nutritional Information:

This recipe makes 4 servings. Each serving contains approximately:

- 400 calories

- 15g fat

- 40g carbohydrates

- 14g protein

- 5g fiber

Variations:

- Gluten-free: Use gluten-free lentils and ensure all ingredients are gluten-free.

- Dairy-free: Omit the cheese or use a dairy-free alternative.

- Vegan: Omit the cheese and use a vegan-friendly balsamic vinegar.

- Vegetarian: Follow the vegan variation and add cooked shrimp or fish to the salad.

- Keto: Omit the peas and use a low-carb vegetable broth.

- Pescetarian: Add cooked shrimp or fish to the salad.

- Lactose-free: Use a lactose-free vegetable broth.

Serving Tip:

Garnish with diced scallions and serve with a side of brown rice or quinoa for a complete meal.

Bonus Health Tip:

Spinach is a great source of vitamins and minerals, including vitamin A, vitamin C, and folate, which are essential for thyroid function. Incorporating spinach into your diet can help prevent hypothyroidism and promote overall health. Try adding spinach to your smoothies, salads, or sautéed dishes for a healthy and delicious treat.

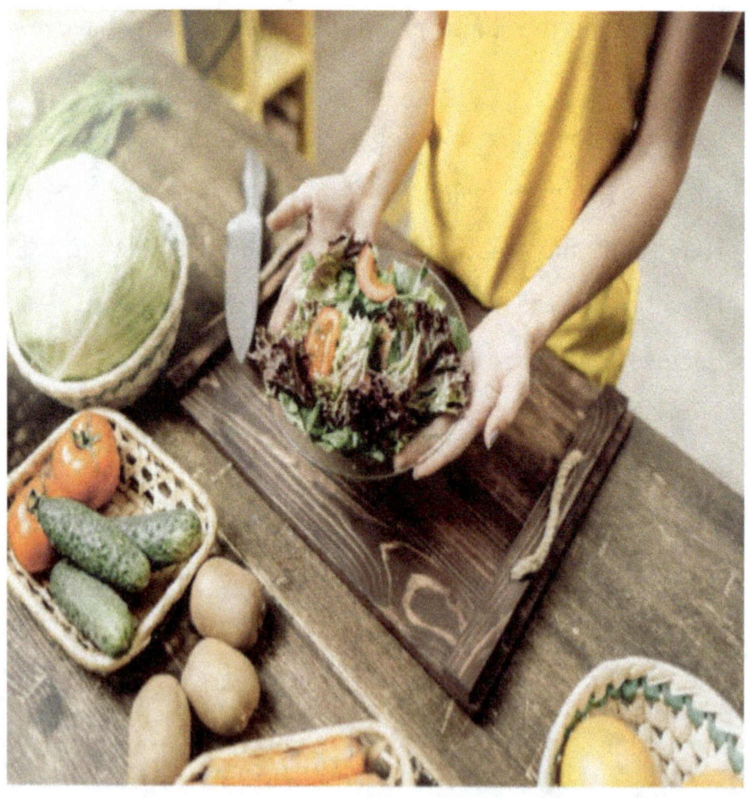

CHAPTER 3

Wholesome Main Courses

When it comes to maintaining a healthy lifestyle, the food we eat plays a crucial role. In Chapter 3 of our journey through hypothyroidism, we will explore the significance of wholesome main courses in managing this condition. From nutrient-dense ingredients to delicious recipes, this chapter will guide you in making informed and delectable choices to support your well-being. So, let's embark on this culinary adventure together, discovering the power of wholesome eating in the context of hypothyroidism.

- Lemon-Herb Baked Salmon

Looking for a delicious and healthy recipe that can help manage hypothyroidism? Look no further than Lemon-Herb Baked Salmon! This recipe is packed with ingredients that are beneficial for thyroid function, including salmon, which is rich in omega-3 fatty acids, and herbs, which are a great source of vitamins and minerals. The recipe is simple and easy to follow, and can be adapted to meet different dietary needs, such as gluten-free, dairy-free, vegan, or vegetarian. Here's how to make it:

Ingredients:

- 4 salmon filets

- 2 tbsp melted butter

- 2 tbsp chopped fresh parsley

- 2 tbsp chopped fresh basil

- 2 tbsp chopped fresh rosemary

- 1 clove garlic, minced

- 1 lemon, juiced and zested

- Salt and pepper, to taste

Instructions:

1. Preheat the oven to 400°F.

2. In a small bowl, mix together the melted butter, chopped herbs, minced garlic, lemon juice, and lemon zest.

3. Place the salmon filets skin-side down in a baking dish.

4. Brush the herb mixture over the salmon filets.

5. Season it with salt and pepper to taste.

6. Bake for 15-20 minutes, or until the salmon is cooked through.

7. Serve immediately.

Nutritional Information:

This recipe makes 4 servings. Each serving contains approximately:

- 350 calories

- 20g fat

- 2g carbohydrates

- 38g protein

- 1g fiber

Variations:

- Gluten-free: Ensure all ingredients are gluten-free.

- Dairy-free: Use a dairy-free butter alternative.

- Vegan: Use a vegan butter alternative and substitute the salmon with a vegan protein source, such as tofu or tempeh.

- Vegetarian: Follow the vegan variation and add cheese or eggs for additional protein.

- Keto: Omit the lemon juice and use a low-carb butter alternative.

- Pescetarian: Follow the original recipe.

Serving Tip:

Serve with a side of roasted vegetables, such as asparagus or brussels sprouts, for a complete meal.

Bonus Health Tip:

Salmon is a great source of omega-3 fatty acids, which are essential for thyroid function. Incorporating salmon into your diet can help prevent hypothyroidism and promote overall health. Try adding salmon to your diet at least once a week for a healthy and delicious treat.

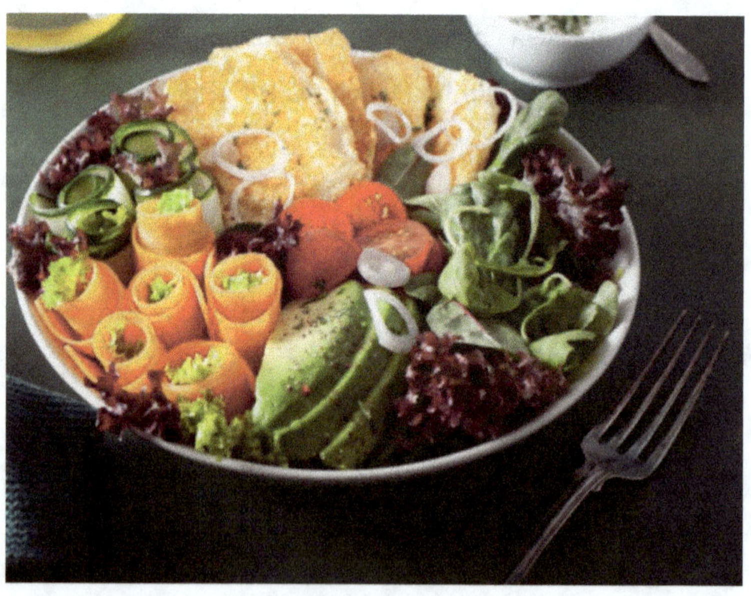

- Turkey and Quinoa Stuffed Peppers

Looking for a delicious and healthy recipe that can help heal hypothyroidism? Look no further than Turkey and Quinoa Stuffed Peppers! This recipe is packed with ingredients that are beneficial for thyroid function, including ground turkey, which is a great source of protein, and quinoa, which is a great source of fiber and minerals. The recipe is simple and easy to follow, and can be adapted to meet different dietary needs, such as gluten-free, dairy-free, vegan, or vegetarian. Here's how to make it:

Ingredients:

- 4-5 bell peppers, preferred color

- 1/2 cup uncooked quinoa

- 1 cup water

- 1/2 cup red onion, chopped

- 1 lb ground turkey

- 1 cup tomato sauce or marinara sauce (either is fine)

- 1 tablespoon Italian seasoning

- Optional add-on: Parmesan cheese

Instructions:

1. Preheat the oven to 375°F.

2. In a deep skillet, begin to sauté the ground turkey and red onion. When the turkey has started to turn brown, add in the cooked quinoa along with tomato sauce and 1 tablespoon Italian seasoning. Continue to cook the mixture for about 5-10 minutes.

3. While the turkey quinoa mixture is cooking, cut the tops off of each bell pepper and remove all the seeds. Then place the bell peppers on a baking dish.

4. As soon as the turkey quinoa mixture has finished cooking, carefully spoon it into each of the bell peppers. Fill each pepper all the way to the top.

5. Sprinkle Parmesan cheese on top of each pepper.

6. Bake for 30-35 minutes, or until the peppers are tender and the cheese is melted.

7. Serve immediately.

Nutritional Information:

This recipe makes 4-5 servings. Each serving contains approximately:

- 300-350 calories

- 10-15g fat

- 20-25g carbohydrates

- 25-30g protein

- 5-7g fiber

Variations:

- Gluten-free: Use gluten-free quinoa and ensure all ingredients are gluten-free.

- Dairy-free: Omit the cheese or use a dairy-free alternative.

- Vegan: Omit the cheese and substitute the ground turkey with a vegan protein source, such as tofu or tempeh.

- Vegetarian: Follow the vegan variation and add cheese or eggs for additional protein.

- Keto: Omit the quinoa and use a low-carb vegetable, such as cauliflower rice, instead.

- Pescetarian: Substitute the ground turkey with cooked shrimp or fish.

- Lactose-free: Use a lactose-free tomato sauce.

Serving Tip:

Garnish with chopped fresh herbs, such as parsley or basil, for added flavor and nutrition.

Bonus Health Tip:

Quinoa is a great source of fiber and minerals, including magnesium and zinc, which are essential for thyroid function. Incorporating quinoa into your diet can help prevent hypothyroidism and promote overall health. Try adding quinoa to your salads, soups, or stir-fry dishes for a healthy and delicious treat.

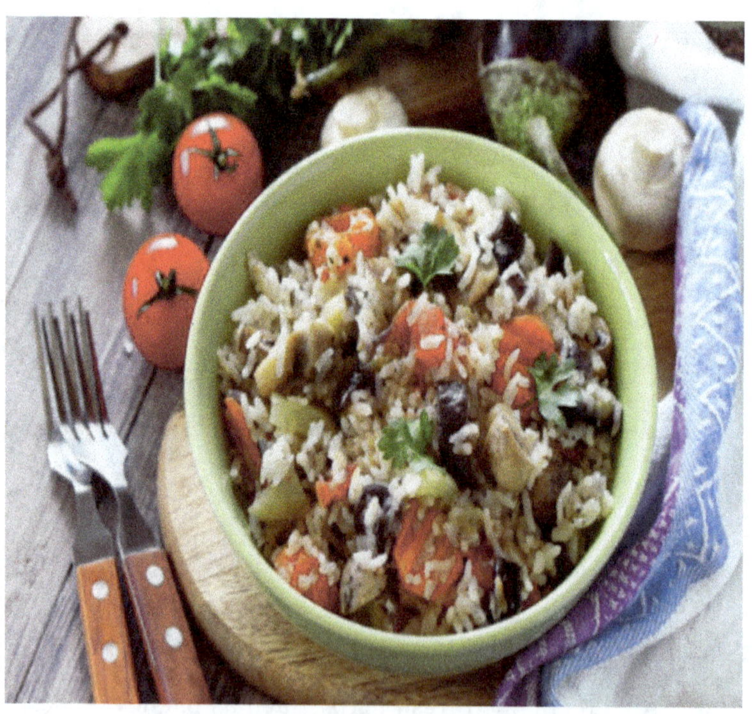

- Chickpea Curry Delight

Are you looking for a delicious and nutritious Chickpea Curry that can help manage hypothyroidism? Look no further than Chickpea Curry Delight! This recipe is packed with ingredients that are beneficial for thyroid function, including chickpeas, which are rich in protein and fiber, and a blend of spices that are known to support overall health. The recipe is simple and easy to follow, and can be adapted to meet different dietary needs, such as gluten-free, dairy-free, vegan, or vegetarian. Here's how to make it:

Ingredients:

- 2 tablespoons vegetable oil or coconut oil
- 1 medium onion, sliced
- 3 cloves garlic, minced
- ¼ teaspoon crushed red pepper flakes
- 1-2 tablespoons curry powder
- 1 teaspoon ground cumin
- 2 cups of fresh or canned diced tomatoes
- 3 cups cooked chickpeas
- 13.5 ounces canned coconut milk
- Salt and pepper, to taste

- Optional garnishes: chopped cilantro, julienned ginger, and a squeeze of lemon juice

Instructions:

1. In a large pot or Dutch oven, heat the vegetable oil or coconut oil over medium heat.

2. Add the onion and cook for about 5 minutes until softened

3. Add the garlic and red pepper flakes, and cook for an additional 1-2 minutes, until fragrant.

4. Stir in the curry powder and ground cumin, and cook for about 1 minute, until the spices are toasted.

5. Add the diced tomatoes, chickpeas, and coconut milk to the pot. Stir to combine.

6. Bring the mixture to a boil, then reduce the heat to low and let it simmer for 20-30 minutes, or until the sauce has thickened slightly.

7. Season with salt and pepper to taste, and adjust other seasonings as necessary.

8. Serve hot, garnished with chopped cilantro, julienned ginger, and a squeeze of lemon juice, if desired.

Nutritional Information:

This recipe makes 4 servings. Each serving contains approximately:

- 400 calories

- 15g fat

- 20g carbohydrates

- 25g protein

- 5g fiber

Variations:

- Gluten-free: Ensure all ingredients are gluten-free.

- Dairy-free: Use a dairy-free coconut milk alternative or omit the coconut milk and use a dairy-free milk, such as almond or cashew milk.

- Vegan: Omit the coconut milk and use a vegan-friendly milk alternative. Substitute the chickpeas with a vegan protein source, such as tofu or tempeh.

- Vegetarian: Follow the vegan variation and add cheese or eggs for additional protein.

- Keto: Omit the chickpeas and use a low-carb vegetable, such as cauliflower rice, instead.

- Pescetarian: Substitute the chickpeas with cooked shrimp or fish.

- Lactose-free: Use a lactose-free tomato sauce.

Serving Tip:

Garnish with chopped fresh herbs for added flavor and nutrition, such as parsley or cilantro.

Bonus Health Tip:

Chickpeas are a great source of fiber and minerals, including magnesium and zinc, which are essential for thyroid function. Incorporating chickpeas into your diet can help prevent hypothyroidism and promote overall health. Try adding chickpeas to your salads, soups, or stir-fry dishes for a healthy and delicious treat.

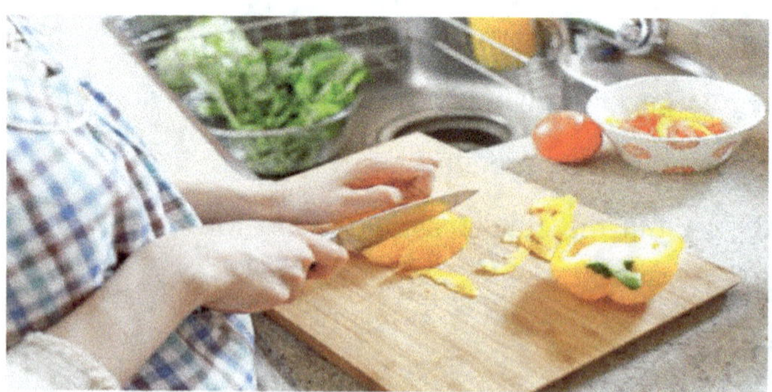

- Herbed Chicken with Sweet Potatoes

This recipe is packed with ingredients that are beneficial for thyroid function, including chicken, sweet potatoes, and a blend of herbs that are known to support overall health. The recipe is simple and easy to follow, and can be adapted to meet different dietary needs, such as gluten-free, dairy-free, vegan, or vegetarian. Here's how to make it:

Ingredients:

- 1 lb boneless skinless chicken breasts, cut into bite-sized pieces
- 2 large peeled and diced sweet potatoes, into 1-inch cubes
- 1 tbsp olive oil
- 1/2 tsp garlic powder
- 1/2 tsp Italian seasoning
- Salt and pepper, to taste
- 1/4 cup chicken broth
- 2 tbsp balsamic vinegar
- 2 tbsp honey
- 1 tbsp fresh lemon juice
- 1 tbsp chopped fresh parsley
- 1 tbsp chopped fresh basil

- 1 tbsp chopped fresh oregano

Instructions:

1. Preheat the oven to 400°F (200°C).

2. In a large bowl, toss the chicken with olive oil, garlic powder, Italian seasoning, salt, and pepper.

3. In a separate bowl, whisk together the chicken broth, balsamic vinegar, honey, and lemon juice.

4. Place the chicken and sweet potatoes on a baking sheet, and pour the honey mixture over the top.

5. Roast in the preheated oven for 20-25 minutes, or until the chicken is cooked through and the sweet potatoes are tender.

6. Remove from the oven and garnish with chopped fresh herbs.

7. Serve immediately.

Nutritional Information:

This recipe makes 4 servings. Each serving contains approximately:

- 300 calories

- 10g fat

- 20g carbohydrates

- 25g protein

- 2g fiber

Variations:

- Gluten-free: Ensure all ingredients are gluten-free.

- Dairy-free: Use a dairy-free honey alternative and omit the cheese or use a dairy-free cheese.

- Vegan: Omit the honey and use a vegan-friendly balsamic vinegar. Substitute the chicken with a vegan protein source, such as tofu or tempeh.

- Vegetarian: Follow the vegan variation and add cheese or eggs for additional protein.

- Keto: Omit the sweet potatoes and use a low-carb protein source, such as fish or tofu.

- Pescetarian: Substitute the chicken with cooked shrimp or fish.

- Lactose-free: Use a lactose-free chicken broth.

Serving Tip:

Garnish with chopped fresh herbs, such as parsley, basil, or oregano, for added flavor and nutrition.

Bonus Health Tip:

Sweet potatoes are a great source of vitamins and minerals, including vitamin A, vitamin C, and vitamin B6, which are essential for thyroid function. Incorporating sweet potatoes into your diet can help prevent hypothyroidism and promote overall health. Try adding sweet potatoes to your soups, salads, or main dishes for a healthy and delicious treat.

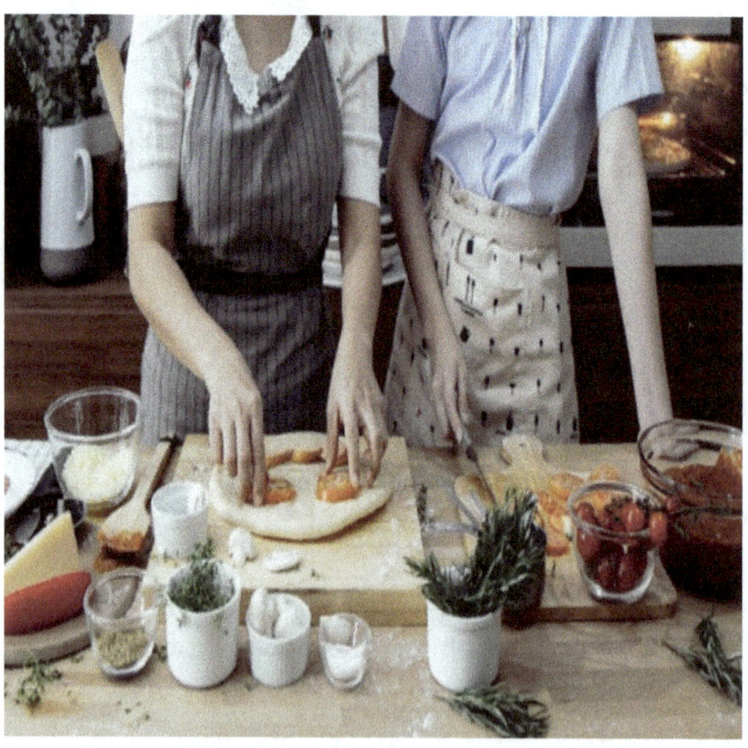

CHAPTER 4

Satisfying Snacks and Sides

Welcome to Chapter 4 of our journey through hypothyroidism, where we explore the world of satisfying snacks and sides. Hypothyroidism is a condition characterized by low thyroid hormone production, which can lead to a range of symptoms and health issues if left untreated. While medication is often necessary to manage this condition, a healthy diet can also play a crucial role in supporting thyroid function and overall well-being. In this chapter, we will delve into the importance of wholesome snacks and sides in the context of hypothyroidism, offering insights into nutrient-rich ingredients and delicious recipes to aid in managing this condition. So, join us on this culinary adventure, where we will discover the power of satisfying and nourishing foods in the context of hypothyroidism.

- Crunchy Kale Chips

These homemade chips are not only irresistibly crispy, but they also offer a wealth of nutrients that can benefit thyroid health. Kale is a fantastic source of vitamins and minerals, while being low in calories and high in fiber. These chips are a great alternative to traditional potato chips, and you won't be able to stop at just one!

Ingredients:

- 1 large bundle curly green or purple kale
- 1-2 Tbsp melted coconut or avocado oil
- Seasonings of choice (i.e. a pinch sea salt, 1 tsp cumin powder, 1 tsp chili powder, 1 tsp curry powder, 1 Tbsp nutritional yeast, etc. / measurements listed per 1 large bundle kale)

Step by Step Instructions:

1. Preheat the oven to 225 degrees F (107 C). Use convection bake if you have it to speed cooking time and help chips crisp up more.
2. Rinse and thoroughly dry kale, next tear into small pieces and discard any large stems.
3. Massage the kale with oil and your choice of seasonings.
4. Spread the kale out on baking sheets, ensuring they touch as little as possible.

5. Bake for 15 minutes, then stir gently and bake a little longer until crispy and very slightly golden brown. Watch carefully to prevent burning!

Nutritional Information:

Kale chips are low in calories and high in nutrients, providing a good dose of vitamins A, K, and C, as well as minerals like calcium and potassium. The exact nutritional content will depend on the specific ingredients and seasonings used.

Variations:

- Gluten-free: Kale chips are naturally gluten-free.

- Dairy-free: Kale chips are naturally dairy-free.

- Vegan: Use plant-based seasonings like nutritional yeast for a cheesy flavor.

- Keto: Kale chips are low in carbs and can be enjoyed on a keto diet.

- Pescetarian: Kale chips are naturally pescetarian-friendly.

Serving Tip:

Enjoy these kale chips on their own as a snack, or pair them with a dip of your choice for added flavor.

Bonus Health Tip:

Kale is a cruciferous vegetable, which means it's high in compounds that support healthy liver function. Since the liver plays a key role in thyroid health, incorporating kale into your diet can be beneficial for those with hypothyroidism.

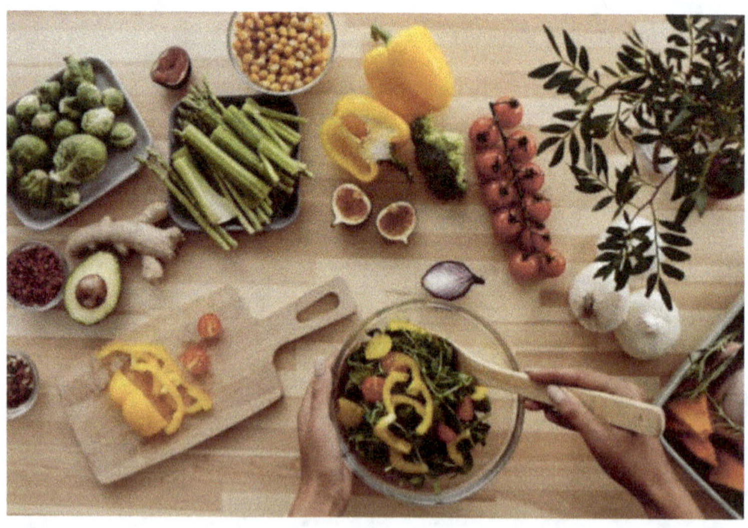

- Hummus Trio (Classic, Beetroot, Spinach)

Looking for a versatile and nutritious snack that can also support your journey to manage hypothyroidism? Indulge in this delightful Hummus Trio, featuring classic, beetroot, and spinach variations. Hummus, a traditional Middle Eastern dip, is a great source of plant-based protein and fiber, both of which are beneficial for thyroid health. The addition of nutrient-dense vegetables like beetroots and spinach further enhances the nutritional profile of this snack, making it a perfect choice for those looking to support their thyroid health.

Ingredients:

- 24 oz (675 g) hummus, divided
- 1 small avocado, sliced
- 3 oz (85 g) red pepper, roasted
- 1/2 cup (100 g) canned beet
- Pita chips, for serving

Step by Step Instructions:

1. In a food processor, combine 8 ounces (225 g) of hummus with the avocado. Puree until smooth. Transfer to a small bowl.

2. Clean the food processor. Add 8 ounces (225 g) of hummus and the red peppers. Puree until smooth. Transfer to another small bowl.

3. Clean the food processor. Add the remaining hummus and the beets. Puree until smooth. Transfer to another small bowl.

4. Serve with pita chips.

5. Enjoy!

Nutritional Information:

- Calories: 143
- Fat: 8g
- Carbs: 12g
- Fiber: 5g
- Sugar: 1g
- Protein: 5g

Variations:

- Gluten-free: Ensure the pita chips are gluten-free.

- Dairy-free: The recipe is naturally dairy-free.

- Vegan: This recipe is vegan-friendly.

- Keto: Enjoy with keto-friendly vegetable sticks instead of pita chips.

- Pescetarian: This recipe is pescetarian-friendly.

Serving Tip:

Pair the hummus trio with an assortment of fresh vegetable sticks, such as carrots, cucumbers, and bell peppers, for a colorful and nutritious snack.

Bonus Health Tip:

Beetroots are rich in nitrates, which can help improve blood flow and support heart health. A healthy cardiovascular system is important for individuals with hypothyroidism, as it can help ensure efficient transport of thyroid hormones throughout the body.

- Oven-Baked Sweet Potato Fries

These oven-baked sweet potato fries are a fantastic alternative to traditional fries. Sweet potatoes are a great source of vitamins and minerals, including vitamin A, which is essential for thyroid health. Baking them in the oven with a touch of olive oil and seasoning makes them a healthier option compared to traditional fries, and they are just as tasty.

Ingredients:

- 2 pounds of sweet potatoes (about 2 medium-large or 3 medium)
- 1 tablespoon cornstarch
- ½ teaspoon fine sea salt
- 2 tablespoons extra-virgin olive oil
- Optional spices: freshly ground black pepper, garlic pepper, and/or cayenne powder

Step by Step Instructions:

1. Preheat the oven to 425 degrees Fahrenheit with racks in the lower and upper thirds of the oven.

2. Peel the sweet potatoes and cut them into fry-shaped pieces about ¼″ wide and ¼″ thick.

3. In a large bowl, toss the sweet potatoes with cornstarch and salt until they are evenly coated.

4. Drizzle the olive oil over the sweet potatoes and toss until they are lightly coated.

5. Arrange the sweet potatoes in a single layer on two rimmed baking sheets.

6. Bake the sweet potatoes, flipping once halfway through, until they are tender and browned, about 25 to 30 minutes.

Nutritional Information:

- Calories: 143

- Fat: 8g

- Carbs: 12g

- Fiber: 5g

- Sugar: 1g

- Protein: 5g

Variations:

- Gluten-free: These sweet potato fries are naturally gluten-free.

- Dairy-free: The recipe is naturally dairy-free.

- Vegan: This recipe is vegan-friendly.

- Keto: Sweet potatoes are not typically consumed on a keto diet due to their higher carb content.

- Pescetarian: This recipe is pescetarian-friendly.

Serving Tip:

Enjoy these sweet potato fries as a side dish or a healthy snack. They pair well with a variety of dipping sauces, such as ketchup, aioli, or a spicy mayo.

Bonus Health Tip:

Sweet potatoes are a great source of beta-carotene, which is converted into vitamin A in the body. Vitamin A is essential for thyroid health and overall well-being.

- Almond and Pumpkin Seed Trail Mix

If you're seeking a nutritious and convenient snack to support your journey in healing hypothyroidism, this almond and pumpkin seed trail mix is an excellent choice. Almonds are a great source of healthy fats and protein, while pumpkin seeds are rich in magnesium and other essential nutrients that can benefit thyroid health. This trail mix is not only delicious but also provides a good balance of nutrients, making it a perfect snack for those looking to support their thyroid health.

Ingredients:

- 1 cup raw almonds
- 1 cup raw pumpkin seeds (pepitas)
- 1-2 tablespoons maple syrup or honey
- 1/2 teaspoon ground cinnamon
- 1/4 teaspoon sea salt
- 1/2 cup dried cranberries or raisins

Step by Step Instructions:

1. Preheat the oven to 325°F (163°C).

2. In a bowl, combine the almonds, pumpkin seeds, maple syrup or honey, cinnamon, and sea salt. Toss until the nuts and seeds are well coated.

3. Spread the mixture in a single layer on a baking sheet lined with parchment paper.

4. Bake for 15-20 minutes, stirring once or twice, until the nuts are golden and the syrup is caramelized.

5. Remove from the oven and let the mixture cool completely.

6. Once cooled, add the dried cranberries or raisins and toss to combine.

7. Store the trail mix in an airtight container.

Nutritional Information:

- Serving size: 1/4 cup

- Calories: 180

- Fat: 14g

- Carbohydrates: 10g

- Fiber: 3g

- Sugar: 5g

- Protein: 7g

Variations:

- Gluten-free: This trail mix is naturally gluten-free.

- Dairy-free: The recipe is naturally dairy-free.

- Vegan: Use maple syrup instead of honey for a vegan-friendly option.

- Keto: Adjust the amount of dried fruit to reduce the carb content for a keto-friendly version.

- Pescetarian: This recipe is pescetarian-friendly.

Serving Tip:

Enjoy this trail mix as an on-the-go snack, or sprinkle it over yogurt or oatmeal for a nutritious boost.

Bonus Health Tip:

Pumpkin seeds are an excellent source of magnesium, which is important for thyroid function. Additionally, the healthy fats and protein from the almonds make this trail mix a great option for supporting overall thyroid health.

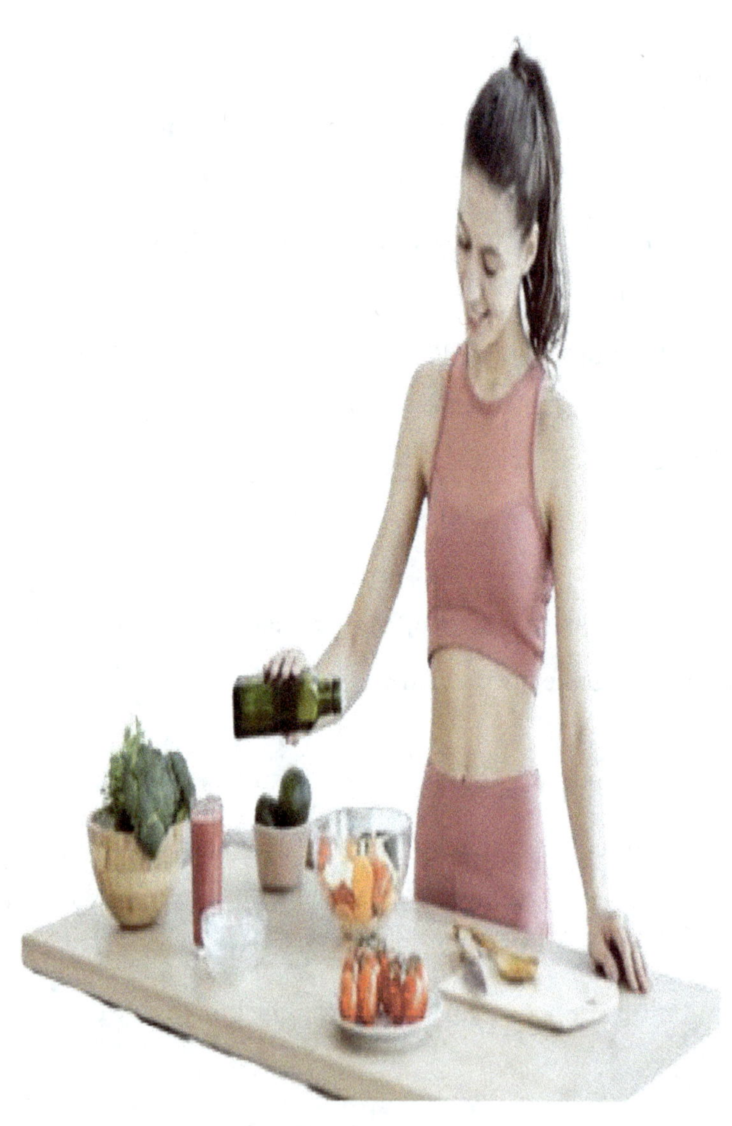

CHAPTER 5

Decadent Desserts (Yes, You Can!)

Let's explore the importance of indulgent desserts in the context of hypothyroidism, offering insights into nutrient-rich ingredients and delicious recipes to aid in managing this condition. So, join us on this culinary adventure, where we will discover the power of satisfying and nourishing foods in the context of hypothyroidism.

- Chocolate Avocado Pudding

This creamy and decadent chocolate avocado pudding is not only a delicious dessert but also a nutritious option for those looking to support their thyroid health. Avocados are a great source of healthy fats and magnesium, which are beneficial for thyroid function. This pudding is easy to make and can be tailored to various dietary needs, making it a versatile and satisfying treat for anyone on a journey to manage hypothyroidism.

Ingredients:

- 2 ripe avocados

- 4 tablespoons unsweetened cocoa powder

- 2-3 tablespoons pure maple syrup

- 1/2 teaspoon vanilla extract

- Pinch of salt

- 2 tablespoons water, or more as needed for you to blend

Step by Step Instructions:

1. Scoop the avocado flesh into a blender or food processor.

2. Add the cocoa powder, maple syrup, vanilla extract, salt, and water.

3. Blend until smooth and creamy, scraping down the sides as needed.

4. If the pudding is too thick, add more water, 1 tablespoon at a time, until it reaches your desired consistency.

5. Taste the pudding and adjust the sweetness or cocoa powder to your preference.

6. Transfer the pudding to serving dishes and chill in the refrigerator for at least 30 minutes before serving.

Nutritional Information:

- Serving size: 1/2 cup

- Calories: 220

- Fat: 15g

- Carbohydrates: 25g

- Fiber: 10g

- Sugar: 10g

- Protein: 3g

Variations:

- Gluten-free: This pudding is naturally gluten-free.

- Dairy-free: The recipe is naturally dairy-free.

- Vegan: This recipe is vegan-friendly.

- Keto: Adjust the amount of maple syrup to reduce the carb content for a keto-friendly version.

- Pescetarian: This recipe is pescetarian-friendly.

Serving Tip:

Serve the chocolate avocado pudding with a dollop of coconut whipped cream and a sprinkle of cocoa nibs for an extra special treat.

Bonus Health Tip:

Avocados are a nutrient-dense food, rich in monounsaturated fats and a good source of fiber, potassium, and vitamins. The healthy fats in avocados can help support the absorption of fat-soluble vitamins, making this pudding a nourishing and satisfying dessert option for those with hypothyroidism.

- Berry Bliss Chia Seed Pudding

This vibrant and delicious berry chia seed pudding is not only a delightful treat but also a nutritious option for those looking to support their thyroid health. Chia seeds are rich in omega-3 fatty acids, fiber, and antioxidants, which can benefit thyroid function. This pudding is easy to make and can be tailored to various dietary needs, making it a versatile and satisfying dessert for anyone on a journey to manage hypothyroidism.

Ingredients:
- 1 1/2 cups mixed berries (fresh or frozen), divided
- 1/4 cup chia seeds
- 1 3/4 cups unsweetened almond milk or other plant-based milk
- 2-3 tablespoons pure maple syrup or honey
- 1 teaspoon vanilla extract
- Pinch of salt

Step by Step Instructions:

1. In a blender or food processor, combine 1 cup of mixed berries, chia seeds, almond milk, maple syrup or honey, vanilla extract, and salt.

2. Blend until smooth and creamy, scraping down the sides as needed.

3. Pour the mixture into a large bowl or container, cover, and refrigerate for at least 1 hour or up to overnight.

4. In the morning, remove the pudding from the refrigerator and let it sit at room temperature for a few minutes.

5. Stir the pudding well to redistribute the chia seeds and berries.

6. Serve the pudding topped with the remaining 1/2 cup of mixed berries.

Nutritional Information:

- Serving size: 1/2 cup

- Calories: 180

- Fat: 14g

- Carbohydrates: 25g

- Fiber: 3g

- Sugar: 10g

- Protein: 3g

Variations:

- Gluten-free: This pudding is naturally gluten-free.

- Dairy-free: The recipe is naturally dairy-free.

- Vegan: This recipe is vegan-friendly.

- Keto: Adjust the amount of maple syrup to reduce the carb content for a keto-friendly version.

- Pescetarian: This recipe is pescetarian-friendly.

Serving Tip:

Serve the berry chia seed pudding with a dollop of Greek yogurt or coconut whipped cream and a sprinkle of granola for an extra special treat.

Bonus Health Tip:

Chia seeds are a great source of omega-3 fatty acids, fiber, and antioxidants, which can help support overall health, including thyroid health. The mixed berries in this pudding also provide essential nutrients that can benefit thyroid function.

- Banana-Oatmeal Cookies

If you're looking for a healthy and delicious treat that can also support your journey to heal hypothyroidism, these banana-oatmeal cookies are the perfect option. Packed with nutritious ingredients, such as ripe bananas and oats, these cookies are not only a delightful snack but also a great source of fiber and essential nutrients that can benefit thyroid health.

Ingredients:
- 1 1/2 cups all-purpose flour
- 3 cups old-fashioned oats
- 1 1/2 teaspoons cinnamon
- 1/4 teaspoon nutmeg
- 1 teaspoon baking soda
- 1 scant teaspoon salt
- 2 sticks (1 cup) unsalted butter, cool but still softened
- 1 cup granulated sugar
- 3/4 cup light brown sugar, packed
- 1 large egg
- 1 teaspoon vanilla extract
- 3 ripe bananas, mashed

- 1/4 cup crushed walnuts

Step by Step Instructions:

1. Preheat the oven to 350°F. Line a baking sheet with parchment paper.

2. In a large bowl, mash the bananas until smooth and pureed.

3. Add the oats and stir until the mixture is well combined.

4. Add the chocolate chips or your favorite mix-ins, then stir again.

5. Drop 1 ½ tablespoon portions of dough onto the baking sheet, then use your fingers to flatten them into a round cookie shape.

6. Bake the banana oatmeal cookies for 13 to 15 minutes. Remove from the oven, let it cool for a few minutes, then enjoy.

Nutritional Information:

- Serving size: 1 cookie

- Calories: 180

- Fat: 8g

- Carbohydrates: 25g

- Fiber: 3g

- Sugar: 10g

- Protein: 3g

Variations:

- Gluten-free: Use gluten-free flour blend and gluten-free oats.

- Dairy-free: Use dairy-free chocolate chips and a plant-based butter substitute.

- Vegan: Use a flax egg as a substitute for the egg.

- Keto: These cookies are not suitable for a keto diet due to the high carbohydrate content.

- Pescetarian: This recipe is pescetarian-friendly.

Serving Tip:

Enjoy these banana-oatmeal cookies as a healthy snack or a delicious dessert. They can also be a great on-the-go breakfast option.

Bonus Health Tip:

Bananas are a great source of potassium, which is essential for thyroid health. Additionally, oats are high in fiber, which can help support a healthy digestive system and overall well-being.

- Coconut Flour Cake with Berries

Coconut flour is a great alternative to traditional flours, as it's gluten-free and rich in fiber, which can benefit thyroid health. The addition of berries provides essential nutrients and antioxidants, making this cake a perfect option for those looking to support their thyroid health.

Ingredients:

- 1 cup coconut flour, sifted

- 1/2 cup almond flour, sifted

- 1/2 teaspoon baking soda

- 1/2 teaspoon Celtic sea salt

- 4 large organic or pasture-raised eggs

- 1/4 cup 100% pure maple syrup

- 1 cup unsweetened, organic, full-fat coconut milk

- 1/4 cup (2 ounces) grass-fed butter (melted)

- 1 teaspoon pure vanilla extract

- 1-1/4 cups organic blueberries, well rinsed

- 1 cup raw walnuts, chopped

- 2 tablespoons coconut sugar

- 2 teaspoons ground cinnamon

Step by Step Instructions:

1. Preheat the oven to 350°F. Grease an 8" x 8" square baking pan.

2. In a large bowl, combine the coconut flour, almond flour, baking soda, and salt.

3. In another bowl, whisk together the eggs, maple syrup, coconut milk, melted butter, and vanilla extract.

4. Add the wet ingredients to the dry ingredients and mix well

5. Gently fold in the blueberries.

6. In a separate bowl, combine the walnuts, coconut sugar, and ground cinnamon.

7. Pour the cake batter into the prepared baking pan and sprinkle the walnut mixture on top.

8. Bake for 30-35 minutes, or until a toothpick inserted into the center comes out clean.

9. Allow the cake to cool down before serving.

Nutritional Information:

- Serving size: 1 slice

- Calories: 180

- Fat: 8g

- Carbohydrates: 25g

- Fiber: 3g

- Sugar: 10g

- Protein: 3g

Variations:

- Gluten-free: This cake is naturally gluten-free.

- Dairy-free: Use unrefined coconut oil instead of butter for a dairy-free option.

- Vegan: Substitute the eggs with flax eggs for a vegan-friendly version.

- Pescetarian: This recipe is pescetarian-friendly.

Serving Tip:

Serve the coconut flour cake with berries as a delightful dessert or a sweet treat for special occasions.

Bonus Health Tip:

Coconut flour is a great source of fiber and healthy fats, which can help support a healthy digestive system and overall well-being. The addition of blueberries provides essential nutrients and antioxidants, making this cake a perfect option for those looking to support their thyroid health.

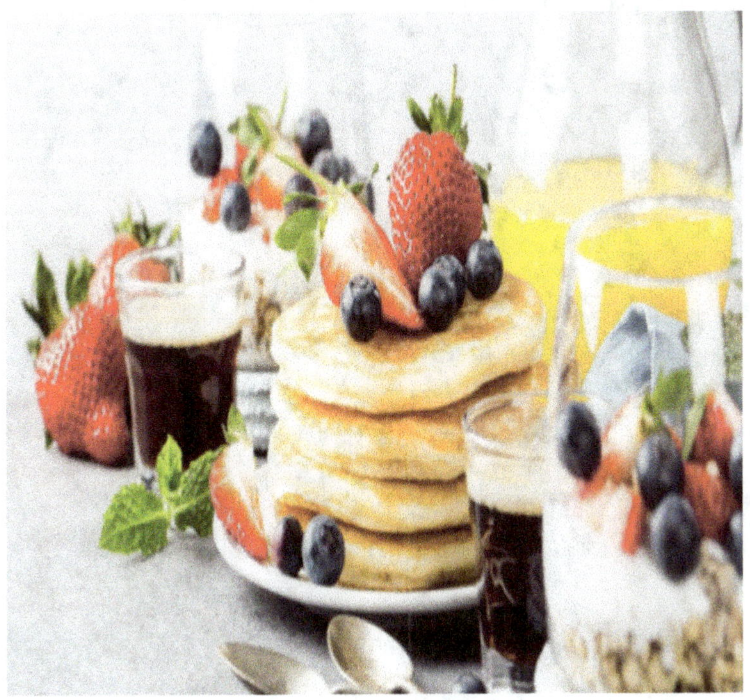

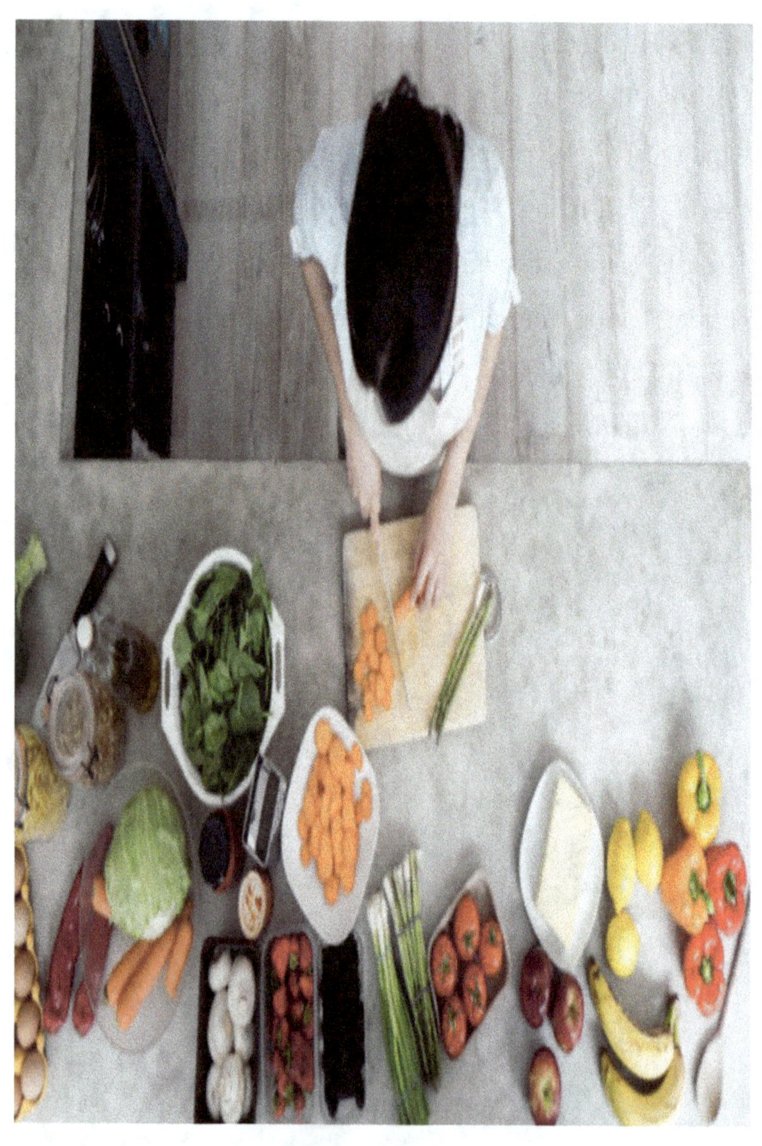

CHAPTER 6

Beverages and Elixirs

In this chapter, we will explore the importance of refreshing beverages and nourishing elixirs in the context of hypothyroidism, offering insights into nutrient-rich ingredients and delicious recipes to aid in managing this condition. So, join us on this culinary adventure, where we will discover the power of satisfying and nourishing foods and drinks in the context of hypothyroidism.

- Thyroid-Boosting Green Tea Elixir

Green tea is a popular beverage that has been shown to have numerous health benefits, including supporting thyroid health. This thyroid-boosting green tea elixir is a delicious and nutritious drink that can help support your journey to heal hypothyroidism. This elixir is made with green tea, which is rich in antioxidants and has been shown to increase metabolism and support weight loss. The addition of other ingredients, such as lemon peel, chamomile, and licorice, makes this elixir a flavorful and nourishing option for those looking to support their thyroid health.

Ingredients:

- 1 green tea bag

- 1 cup boiling water

- 1/2 teaspoon lemon peel

- 1/2 teaspoon chamomile

- 1/2 teaspoon licorice

- 1 teaspoon honey (optional)

Step by Step Instructions:

1. Place the green tea bag in a cup and pour boiling water over it.

2. Add the lemon peel, chamomile, and licorice to the cup.

3. Let the tea steep for 3-5 minutes.

4. Remove the tea bag and strain the tea.

5. Add honey, if desired, and stir well.

6. Enjoy your thyroid-boosting green tea elixir.

Nutritional Information:

- Serving size: 1 cup

- Calories: 5

- Fat: 0g

- Carbohydrates: 1g

- Fiber: 0g

- Sugar: 1g

- Protein: 0g

Variations:

- Gluten-free: This elixir is naturally gluten-free.

- Dairy-free: This recipe is naturally dairy-free.

- Vegan: Substitute maple syrup or agave nectar for honey to make this recipe vegan-friendly.

- Keto: Omit the honey to reduce the carb content for a keto-friendly version.

- Pescetarian: This recipe is pescetarian-friendly.

Serving Tip:

Enjoy this thyroid-boosting green tea elixir as a refreshing and nourishing drink any time of day.

Bonus Health Tip:

Green tea is a great source of antioxidants and has been shown to have numerous health benefits, including supporting thyroid health. The addition of other ingredients, such as lemon peel, chamomile, and licorice, can provide additional benefits, such as reducing inflammation and supporting digestion. Drinking this elixir regularly can be a great way to support your overall health and well-being.

- Berry Antioxidant Smoothie

This berry antioxidant smoothie is a delicious and nutritious drink that can help support your journey to heal hypothyroidism. Packed with antioxidants and essential nutrients, this smoothie is made with a variety of berries, including blueberries, blackberries, and strawberries. These fruits are not only flavorful but also provide numerous health benefits, such as reducing inflammation, lowering blood pressure, and preventing heart disease.

Ingredients:
- 1 cup unsweetened organic coconut water
- 1 1/2 cups fresh or frozen mixed organic berries, such as strawberries, raspberries, and blueberries
- 1/2 cup spinach or kale leaves
- 1/2 cup ice
- 1 tablespoon chia seeds
- 1 tablespoon flax seeds

- 1 tablespoon hemp seeds

- 1 tablespoon maple syrup or honey

Step by Step Instructions:

1. Place the coconut water, berries, spinach or kale leaves, ice, chia seeds, flaxseeds, hemp seeds, and maple syrup or honey in a blender.

2. Blend the ingredients until smooth and creamy.

3. Pour the smoothie into glasses and serve immediately.

Nutritional Information:

- Serving size: 1 cup

- Calories: 150

- Fat: 1g

- Carbohydrates: 25g

- Fiber: 3g

- Sugar: 10g

- Protein: 3g

Variations:

- Gluten-free: This smoothie is naturally gluten-free.

- Dairy-free: This recipe is naturally dairy-free.

- Vegan: Substitute maple syrup or agave nectar for honey to make this recipe vegan-friendly.
- Keto: Omit the maple syrup or agave nectar to reduce the carb content for a keto-friendly version.
- Pescetarian: This recipe is pescetarian-friendly.

Serving Tip:

Enjoy this berry antioxidant smoothie as a refreshing and nourishing drink any time of day.

Bonus Health Tip:

Berries are recognized as some of the most powerful superfoods, providing numerous health benefits. The addition of spinach or kale leaves, chia seeds, flaxseeds, and hemp seeds can further enhance the nutritional value of this smoothie, making it a great option for those looking to support their thyroid health. Drinking this smoothie regularly can be a great way to support your overall health and well-being.

- Golden Milk Latte

The Golden Milk Latte is a warm and comforting beverage that has gained popularity due to its potential health benefits, particularly in supporting thyroid health. This drink is typically made with turmeric, a powerful anti-inflammatory spice, and other warming spices, such as cinnamon and ginger. The addition of black pepper is said to enhance the absorption of curcumin, the active compound in turmeric, making it a great choice for those looking to heal hypothyroidism.

Ingredients:

- 2 cups unsweetened almond milk

- 1/4 teaspoon ground turmeric

- 1/2 inch fresh grated ginger, or 1/8 teaspoon ground ginger

- Pinch of ground cinnamon

- Pinch of black pepper

- 1 teaspoon honey, optional

Step by Step Instructions:

1. In a small saucepan, whisk together the almond milk, turmeric, ginger, cinnamon, and black pepper.

2. Bring the mixture to a simmer over medium heat, whisking frequently.

3. Once the mixture is hot, remove it from the heat and pour it into a mug.

4. Add honey, and stir well, if desired.

5. Serve the golden milk latte immediately.

Nutritional Information:

- Serving size: 1 cup

- Calories: 30

- Fat: 2g

- Carbohydrates: 3g

- Fiber: 1g

- Sugar: 1g

- Protein: 1g

Variations:

- Gluten-free: This golden milk latte is naturally gluten-free.

- Dairy-free: This recipe is naturally dairy-free.

- Vegan: Substitute maple syrup or agave nectar for honey to make this recipe vegan-friendly.

- Keto: Omit the honey to reduce the carb content for a keto-friendly version.

- Pescetarian: This recipe is pescetarian-friendly.

Serving Tip:

Enjoy this golden milk latte as a cozy and nourishing drink any time of day, particularly in the morning or before bed.

Bonus Health Tip:

The turmeric in the golden milk latte is a potent anti-inflammatory and antioxidant, which can help support thyroid health. The addition of warming spices, such as ginger and cinnamon, can also provide additional health benefits, making this drink a great choice for those looking to heal hypothyroidism.

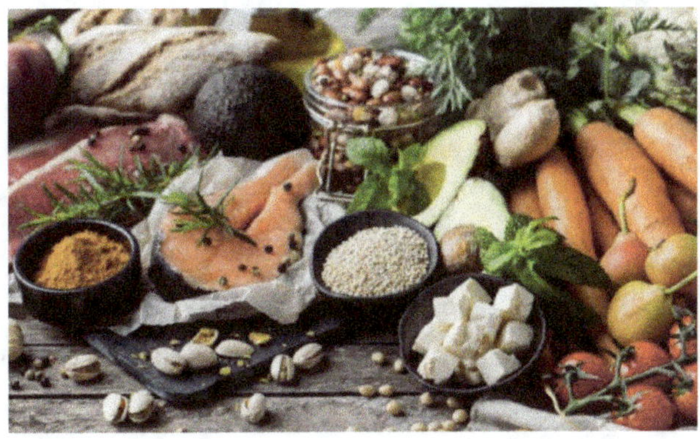

- Refreshing Cucumber Mint Infusion

This refreshing cucumber mint infusion is a hydrating and healthy drink that can help support your journey to heal hypothyroidism. Cucumber is a low-calorie vegetable that is rich in water and electrolytes, making it a great choice for staying hydrated. Mint is a natural digestive aid and can help soothe an upset stomach. This infusion is easy to make and can be customized with other ingredients, such as lemon, lime, or berries, to suit your taste preferences.

Ingredients:

- 1 large cucumber, sliced
- 1/4 cup fresh mint leaves
- 8 cups water
- Optional: lemon or lime slices, berries

Step by Step Instructions:

1. In a large pitcher, combine the sliced cucumber and fresh mint leaves.

2. Add water to the pitcher and stir well.

3. Refrigerate the infusion for at least 1 hour to allow the flavors to meld.

4. Serve the cucumber mint infusion over ice, with optional lemon or lime slices or berries.

Nutritional Information:

- Serving size: 1 cup

- Calories: 0

- Fat: 0g

- Carbohydrates: 0g

- Fiber: 0g

- Sugar: 0g

- Protein: 0g

Variations:

- Gluten-free: This cucumber mint infusion is naturally gluten-free.
- Dairy-free: This recipe is naturally dairy-free.
- Vegan: This recipe is vegan-friendly.
- Keto: This infusion is keto-friendly.
- Pescetarian: This recipe is pescetarian-friendly.

Serving Tip:

Enjoy this refreshing cucumber mint infusion as a hydrating and healthy drink any time of day, particularly during hot weather or after exercise.

Bonus Health Tip:

Staying hydrated is important for overall health and well-being, particularly for those with hypothyroidism. Drinking water and other hydrating beverages, such as this cucumber mint infusion, can help support thyroid function and promote healthy digestion. Adding other ingredients, such as lemon or berries, can provide additional health benefits and make this infusion even more flavorful.

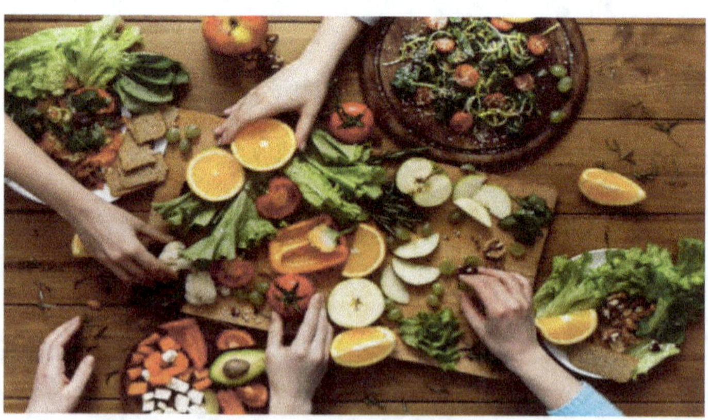

CHAPTER 7

Meal Plans and Tips

This chapter will provide valuable insights into crafting effective meal plans and practical tips to support individuals with hypothyroidism, helping to navigate the complexities of this condition and optimize overall well-being. Join us as we unravel the significance of tailored meal planning and actionable advice in the context of hypothyroidism.

- Weekly Meal Plans for Optimal Thyroid Health

Week 1 Meal Plan

Day 1:

Breakfast: Greek yogurt parfait with mixed berries and a sprinkle of pumpkin seeds.

Lunch: Quinoa salad with roasted vegetables and a side of steamed broccoli.

Dinner: Baked salmon with a quinoa pilaf and sautéed spinach.

Day 2:

Breakfast: Oatmeal topped with sliced banana, walnuts, and a drizzle of honey.

Lunch: Turkey and avocado wrap with whole-grain tortilla and a side of mixed greens.

Dinner: Grilled chicken breast with sweet potato mash and roasted Brussels sprouts.

Day 3:

Breakfast: Spinach and feta omelet with a side of whole-grain toast.

Lunch: Lentil soup with a kale and quinoa salad.

Dinner: Stir-fried tofu with brown rice and mixed vegetables.

Day 4:

Breakfast: Chia seed pudding made with almond milk, topped with sliced strawberries and almonds.

Lunch: Tuna salad with mixed greens and a side of roasted chickpeas.

Dinner: Turkey meatballs served with zucchini noodles and marinara sauce.

Day 5:

Breakfast: Smoothie with spinach, banana, almond butter, and unsweetened almond milk.

Lunch: Grilled vegetable and hummus sandwich on whole-grain bread.

Dinner: Baked cod with quinoa tabbouleh and steamed asparagus.

Day 6:

Breakfast: Whole-grain toast with smashed avocado and a poached egg.

Lunch: Chicken and vegetable stir-fry with brown rice.

Dinner: Beef or tempeh tacos in lettuce wraps with a side of black beans and roasted corn.

Day 7:

Breakfast: Cottage cheese with sliced peaches and a sprinkle of sunflower seeds.

Lunch: Spinach and chickpea salad with grilled chicken.

Dinner: Roasted vegetable medley (bell peppers, onions, tomatoes) with quinoa and a side of grilled shrimp.

Week 2 Meal Plan

Day 1:

Breakfast: Overnight oats with almond milk, sliced apples, and a sprinkle of cinnamon.

Lunch: Grilled chicken salad with mixed greens, cherry tomatoes, and a vinaigrette dressing.

Dinner: Baked halibut with quinoa and roasted vegetables (bell peppers, zucchini, and carrots).

Day 2:

Breakfast: Smoothie with kale, pineapple, Greek yogurt, and a touch of honey.

Lunch: Whole-grain pasta salad with pesto, cherry tomatoes, and grilled shrimp.

Dinner: Turkey chili with black beans, served with a side of steamed broccoli.

Day 3:

Breakfast: Whole-grain toast topped with ricotta cheese, sliced strawberries, and a drizzle of honey.

Lunch: Lentil and vegetable stew with a side of whole-grain bread.

Dinner: Baked chicken thighs with roasted sweet potatoes and sautéed spinach.

Day 4:

Breakfast: Greek yogurt smoothie with mixed berries and a tablespoon of flaxseeds.

Lunch: Tuna and white bean salad with arugula and a lemon vinaigrette.

Dinner: Quinoa-stuffed bell peppers with a side of roasted cauliflower.

Day 5:

Breakfast: Scrambled eggs with spinach and mushrooms, served with whole-grain toast.

Lunch: Grilled vegetable wrap with hummus in a whole-grain tortilla.

Dinner: Baked salmon with quinoa pilaf and steamed asparagus.

Day 6:

Breakfast: Chia seed pudding with almond milk, topped with sliced banana and almonds.

Lunch: Chicken and vegetable stir-fry with brown rice.

Dinner: Beef or tempeh tacos in lettuce wraps with a side of black beans and roasted corn.

Day 7:

Breakfast: Cottage cheese with sliced peaches and a sprinkle of pumpkin seeds.

Lunch: Spinach and chickpea salad with grilled chicken.

Dinner: Grilled shrimp skewers with a quinoa and roasted vegetable medley.

Week 3 Meal Plan

Day 1:

Breakfast: Spinach and tomato omelet with a side of whole-grain toast.

Lunch: Quinoa and black bean salad with diced avocado and a lime vinaigrette.

Dinner: Baked chicken breast with wild rice pilaf and roasted Brussels sprouts.

Day 2:

Breakfast: Greek yogurt parfait with mixed berries and a sprinkle of hemp seeds.

Lunch: Lentil soup with a side of mixed greens and a whole-grain roll.

Dinner: Grilled salmon with quinoa tabbouleh and steamed asparagus.

Day 3:

Breakfast: Overnight oats made with almond milk, topped with sliced peaches and chopped almonds.

Lunch: Turkey and vegetable wrap with hummus in a whole-grain tortilla.

Dinner: Baked tofu with brown rice and a side of sautéed kale.

Day 4:

Breakfast: Whole-grain toast with smashed avocado and a poached egg.

Lunch: Spinach and feta quinoa salad with grilled chicken.

Dinner: Turkey meatballs served with zucchini noodles and marinara sauce.

Day 5:

Breakfast: Smoothie with kale, banana, almond butter, and unsweetened almond milk.

Lunch: Grilled vegetable and quinoa salad with a lemon-herb dressing.

Dinner: Baked cod with sweet potato mash and roasted Brussels sprouts.

Day 6:

Breakfast: Chia seed pudding made with coconut milk, topped with mixed berries and shredded coconut.

Lunch: Chicken and vegetable stir-fry with brown rice.

Dinner: Beef or tempeh tacos in lettuce wraps with a side of black beans and roasted corn.

Day 7:

Breakfast: Cottage cheese with sliced mango and a sprinkle of sunflower seeds.

Lunch: Arugula and chickpea salad with grilled shrimp and a balsamic vinaigrette.

Dinner: Roasted vegetable medley (bell peppers, onions, tomatoes) with quinoa and a side of grilled chicken.

Week 4 Meal Plan

Day 1:

Breakfast: Overnight oats with almond milk, mixed berries, and a sprinkle of chia seeds.

Lunch: Quinoa salad with roasted vegetables (eggplant, bell peppers, and onions) and a side of steamed broccoli.

Dinner: Baked salmon with a side of wild rice and sautéed spinach.

Day 2:

Breakfast: Spinach and feta omelet with whole-grain toast.

Lunch: Lentil soup with a kale and quinoa salad.

Dinner: Grilled chicken breast with sweet potato mash and roasted Brussels sprouts.

Day 3:

Breakfast: Greek yogurt parfait with sliced peaches and a drizzle of honey.

Lunch: Turkey and avocado wrap with whole-grain tortilla and a side of mixed greens.

Dinner: Baked tofu with quinoa and roasted vegetables (zucchini, carrots, and bell peppers).

Day 4:

Breakfast: Chia seed pudding made with almond milk, topped with sliced banana and almonds.

Lunch: Tuna salad with mixed greens and a side of roasted chickpeas.

Dinner: Turkey meatballs served with zucchini noodles and marinara sauce.

Day 5:

Breakfast: Smoothie with kale, pineapple, Greek yogurt, and a touch of honey.

Lunch: Grilled vegetable and hummus sandwich on whole-grain bread.

Dinner: Baked cod with quinoa tabbouleh and steamed asparagus.

Day 6:

Breakfast: Whole-grain toast with smashed avocado and a poached egg.

Lunch: Chicken and vegetable stir-fry with brown rice.

Dinner: Beef or tempeh tacos in lettuce wraps with a side of black beans and roasted corn.

Day 7:

Breakfast: Cottage cheese with sliced strawberries and a sprinkle of pumpkin seeds.

Lunch: Spinach and chickpea salad with grilled chicken.

Dinner: Roasted vegetable medley (bell peppers, onions, tomatoes) with quinoa and a side of grilled shrimp.

- Cooking and Eating Strategies for Managing Hypothyroidism

Managing hypothyroidism through diet is essential for maintaining overall health and well-being. Here are some cooking and eating strategies to help you manage your condition effectively:

1. Focus on nutrient-dense foods: Incorporate whole, nutrient-dense foods like vegetables, fruits, nuts, and fish into your diet. These foods provide essential nutrients such as iodine, selenium, and zinc, which can help maintain a healthy thyroid function.

2. Avoid goitrogens: Goitrogens are compounds found in certain foods that can interfere with thyroid health. However, consuming these foods in moderation does not interfere with overall health and can provide beneficial nutrients.

3. Choose high-quality protein sources: Opt for high-quality protein sources like fish, eggs, and lean meats to support thyroid function.

4. Include healthy fats and carbohydrates: Include moderate amounts of healthy fats and carbohydrates in your diet, such as avocados, nuts, seeds, and whole grains.

5. Stay hydrated: Drinking enough water is crucial for overall health and can help support thyroid function.

6. Meal planning and preparation: Plan your meals in advance and prepare them in bulk to save time and ensure you have nutrient-rich options available.

7. Consider a gluten-free diet: Trialing a gluten-free diet, especially if you have Hashimoto's, can help reduce inflammation and support thyroid health.

8. Monitor your progress: Keep track of how your symptoms and energy levels change as you implement these dietary changes. Adjust your meal plan as needed to optimize your thyroid health.

9. Work with a professional: Consult with a registered dietitian or healthcare professional to develop a personalized meal plan that suits your unique needs and health conditions.

By following these cooking and eating strategies, you can effectively manage your hypothyroidism and support your overall health and well-being.

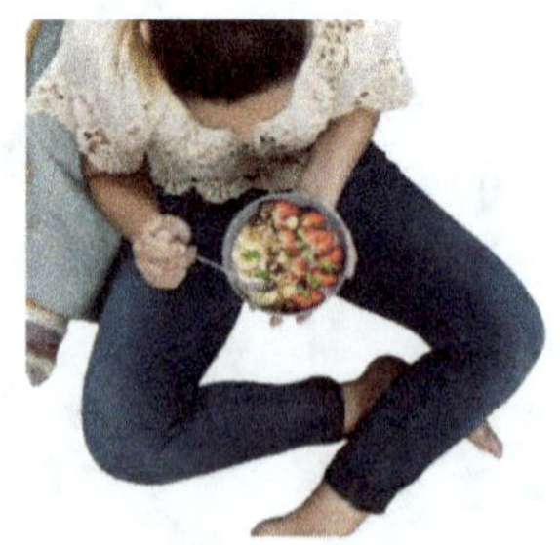

- Ingredient Substitutions and Allergy-Friendly Options

When managing hypothyroidism, ingredient substitutions and allergy-friendly options play a crucial role in maintaining a healthy diet. Below are some strategies and options to consider:

Ingredient Substitutions

1. Beans and Lentils: Chickpeas, kidney beans, or lentils are excellent alternatives for individuals with hypothyroidism, providing a good source of plant-based protein and fiber.

2. Dairy and Nondairy Substitutes: Coconut milk, cashew milk, coconut yogurt, almond milk, and unsweetened yogurt or cheese are suitable replacements for those with dairy sensitivities or following a dairy-free diet.

3. Spices, Herbs, and Condiments: Opt for spices like paprika, saffron, or turmeric, and fresh or dried herbs like basil or rosemary as flavorful alternatives to condiments for individuals with specific dietary restrictions.

Allergy-Friendly Options

1. Gluten-Free Diet: Some individuals with hypothyroidism may benefit from a gluten-free diet, especially those with Hashimoto's disease. This can help reduce inflammation and support thyroid health.

2. Dairy-Free Diet: For individuals with dairy sensitivities or lactose intolerance, dairy-free alternatives such as coconut milk, cashew milk, and almond milk can be used in place of cow's milk in recipes.

3. Plant-Based Milk Substitutes: Options like almond milk, rice milk, and hemp milk can serve as allergy-friendly alternatives to traditional cow's milk for those with dairy or lactose intolerances.

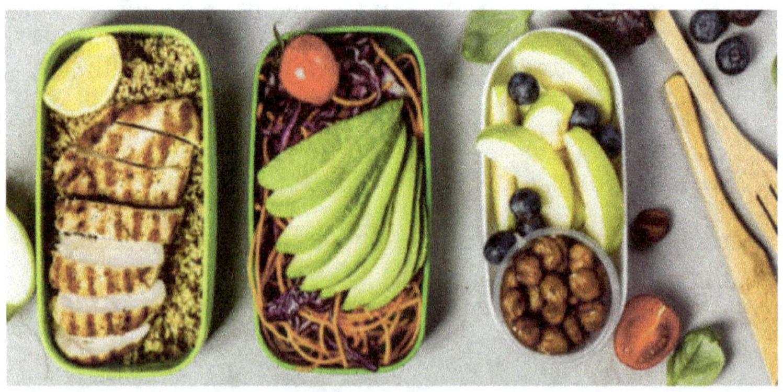

Meal Planning and Preparation

When incorporating these substitutions and allergy-friendly options into your diet, it's important to plan and prepare meals thoughtfully. Consider working with a registered dietitian to develop a balanced eating plan that meets your specific dietary needs and restrictions.

By being mindful of ingredient substitutions and allergy-friendly options, individuals with hypothyroidism can create a varied and nutritious diet that supports their overall health and well-being. Always consult with a healthcare professional or registered dietitian before making significant changes to your diet, especially if you have a pre-existing medical condition or food allergies.

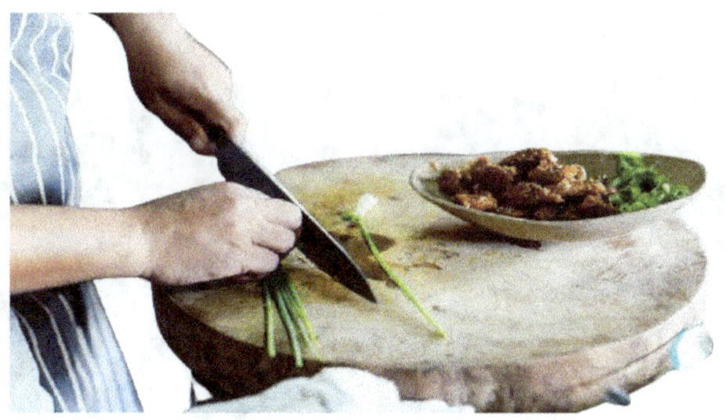

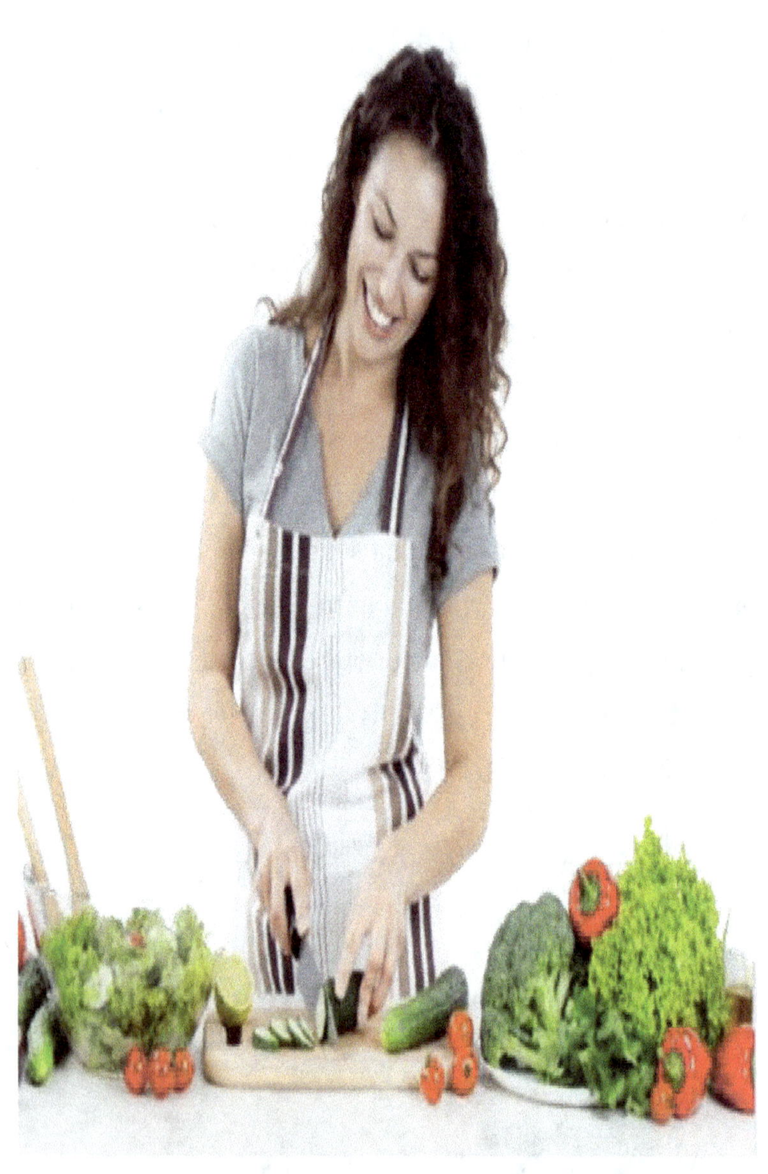

CONCLUSION

- Building a Healthier Lifestyle with Hypothyroidism

Navigating a lifestyle with hypothyroidism can be a journey of self-discovery, resilience, and most importantly, empowerment. Your kitchen becomes not just a space for meal preparation but a sanctuary for nurturing your body and supporting your thyroid health.

Building a healthier lifestyle while managing hypothyroidism begins with understanding the profound impact food choices can have on your well-being. Incorporating nutrient-dense, thyroid-supportive foods lays the foundation for optimal health. From the vibrant colors of fruits and vegetables to the richness of lean proteins and the vitality of whole grains, your choices can make a meaningful difference.

But beyond the ingredients lies the heart of it all—empowerment. Empowerment to experiment with flavors, to craft meals that resonate with your taste buds and nourish your body. It's about forging a positive relationship with food—one that celebrates both pleasure and health.

In your kitchen, armed with knowledge and a commitment to your well-being, you've established a stronghold against the challenges of hypothyroidism. Meal planning, the careful selection of ingredients, and the creativity woven into your culinary endeavors become your tools for embracing a life that thrives despite the condition.

Remember, this journey is unique to you. What works for one may not work for another. Tailor your choices to suit your body's signals and your personal preferences. Seek guidance from healthcare professionals and specialists who can offer personalized advice to complement your journey.

As you continue your kitchen journey, may it be a source of nourishment, joy, and strength. Every meal prepared with care is not just sustenance but a testament to your commitment to thriving with hypothyroidism. You're not just cooking; you're crafting a lifestyle that champions your health and well-being—one meal at a time.

Thank you immensely for choosing "Hypothyroidism Cookbook" as your guide toward healthier eating and well-being. Your support fuels my passion for creating resources that make a difference. Your reviews and feedback mean a lot; they not only assist others but also drive me to keep improving.

If you found this book beneficial, I kindly ask you to leave a review and recommend it to anyone else who might benefit from its insights. Your advocacy helps spread awareness and support to those in need. Thank you for being part of this incredible journey toward better health!

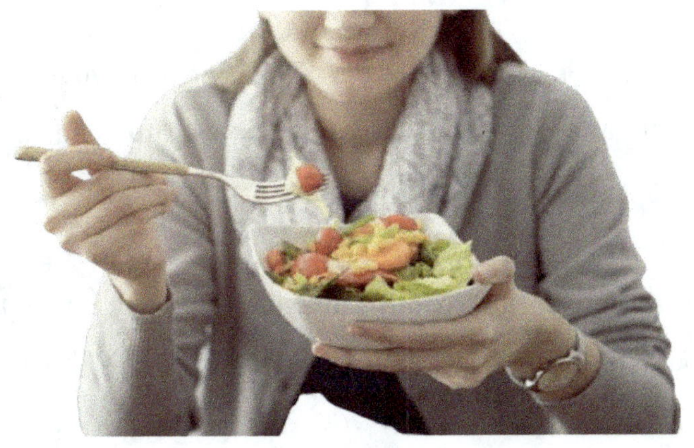

Congratulations on securing your copy of our amazing hypothyroidism cookbook! As a token of our appreciation, you've unlocked a fantastic bonus package:

Guide on Understanding Food Labels for Thyroid-Friendly Ingredients: Dive into this treasure trove of knowledge to decipher labels like a pro! Uncover the best ingredients for supporting your thyroid health.

Thyroid Q&A: Unraveling the Mysteries of Hypothyroidism: Have burning questions? Get ready for an enlightening journey as we demystify the ins and outs of hypothyroidism!

Fun Way to Think About It: Think of it as your secret arsenal - armed with the wisdom to shop smarter and unlock the mysteries of your thyroid health!

Fun Fact about Hypothyroidism: Did you know that hypothyroidism affects more women than men? About 5 to

8 times more women have this condition. Empower yourself with knowledge to conquer this journey to optimal health!

Enjoy your bonus content and happy cooking!

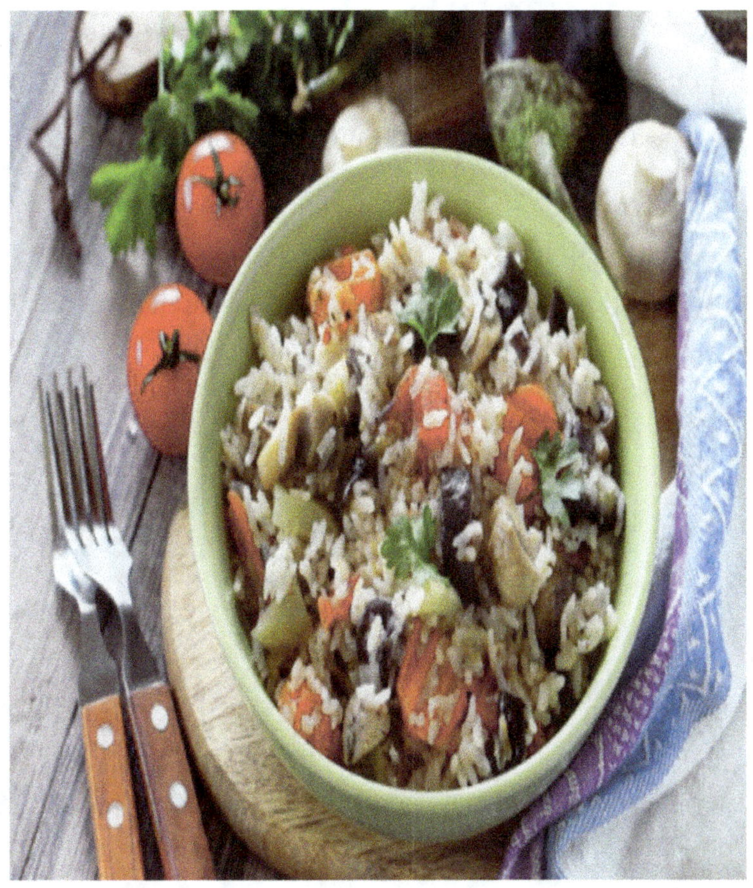

GUIDE ON UNDERSTANDING FOOD LABELS FOR THYROID-FRIENDLY INGREDIENTS

Understanding food labels is crucial for individuals with hypothyroidism who want to make informed dietary choices. Here are some tips for reading food labels to identify thyroid-friendly ingredients:

1. Check for iodine content: Iodine is an essential nutrient for thyroid health, and individuals with hypothyroidism may need to increase their intake of iodine-rich foods. Look for foods that are labeled as a good source of iodine, such as seafood, dairy products, and iodized salt.

2. Avoid goitrogens: Goitrogens are compounds found in certain foods that can interfere with thyroid health. Look for foods that are labeled as goitrogen-free or low in goitrogens, such as kale, spinach, and broccoli.

3. Check for gluten content: Some individuals with hypothyroidism may benefit from a gluten-free diet, especially those with Hashimoto's disease. Look for foods that are labeled as gluten-free, such as gluten-free bread, pasta, and cereals.

4. Avoid artificial sweeteners: Artificial sweeteners like aspartame and sucralose can interfere with thyroid function. Look for foods that are labeled as free from artificial sweeteners or use natural sweeteners like stevia or honey.

5. Check for nutrient content: Look for foods that are high in essential nutrients like selenium, zinc, and vitamin D, which are important for thyroid health. Check the nutrition label to see if the food contains these nutrients.

By being mindful of these tips when reading food labels, individuals with hypothyroidism can make informed dietary choices that support their thyroid health and overall well-being. Remember to consult with a healthcare professional or registered dietitian before making significant changes to your diet, especially if you have a pre-existing medical condition or food allergies.

Understanding food labels is an essential skill for individuals with hypothyroidism who want to make informed dietary choices. By checking for iodine content, avoiding goitrogens and artificial sweeteners, checking for gluten content, and checking for nutrient content, individuals with hypothyroidism can identify thyroid-friendly ingredients and make healthy choices that support their thyroid health.

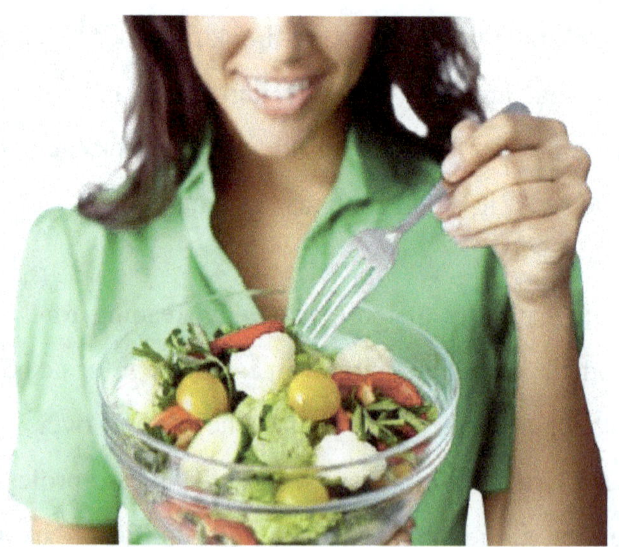

"THYROID Q&A: UNRAVELING THE MYSTERIES OF HYPOTHYROIDISM"

1. What is hypothyroidism?

Hypothyroidism is a condition characterized by low thyroid hormone production, which can lead to a range of symptoms and health issues if left untreated.

2. How does diet affect hypothyroidism?

Diet plays a crucial role in supporting thyroid function and overall well-being in individuals with hypothyroidism.

3. What are some foods to avoid with hypothyroidism?

Individuals with hypothyroidism should avoid goitrogens, which are compounds found in certain foods that can interfere with thyroid health.

4. What are some foods to eat with hypothyroidism?

Individuals with hypothyroidism should focus on consuming a healthy and balanced diet rich in fruits, vegetables, filling proteins, and healthy fats.

5. What is the best diet for hypothyroidism?

The best diet for hypothyroidism is one that is rich in nutrient-dense foods, including iodine-rich seafood, fiber-rich vegetables, and healthy fats.

6. Can a gluten-free diet help manage hypothyroidism?

Some individuals with hypothyroidism may benefit from a gluten-free diet, especially those with Hashimoto's disease.

7. What are some iodine-rich foods?

Iodine-rich foods include seafood, dairy products, and iodized salt.

8. What are some nutrient-rich foods for hypothyroidism?

Nutrient-rich foods for hypothyroidism include selenium-rich foods like Brazil nuts, zinc-rich foods like oysters, and vitamin D-rich foods like fatty fish.

9. Can hypothyroidism cause weight gain?

Yes, hypothyroidism can cause weight gain due to a slowed metabolism.

10. What are some weight loss tips for individuals with hypothyroidism?

Weight loss tips for individuals with hypothyroidism include consuming a healthy and balanced diet, engaging in regular exercise, and managing stress levels.

11. Can certain nutrients interfere with thyroid health?

Yes, certain nutrients like goitrogens and artificial sweeteners can interfere with thyroid health.

12. What are some healthy fats for hypothyroidism?

Healthy fats for hypothyroidism include avocados, nuts, seeds, and fatty fish.

13. Can hypothyroidism be managed through diet alone?

While medication is often necessary to manage hypothyroidism, a healthy diet can also play a crucial role in supporting thyroid function and overall well-being.

14. What are some ingredient substitutions for individuals with hypothyroidism?

Ingredient substitutions for individuals with hypothyroidism include using beans and lentils as a protein source and coconut milk or almond milk as a dairy substitute.

15. Can hypothyroidism be cured through diet?

While changing the diet cannot cure hypothyroidism, it can help manage the condition and improve quality of life.

16. What are some gluten-free grains for individuals with hypothyroidism?

Gluten-free grains for individuals with hypothyroidism include quinoa, rice, and buckwheat.

17. Can iodine supplements help manage hypothyroidism?

Iodine supplements should only be taken under the guidance of a healthcare professional, as excessive iodine intake can be harmful to thyroid health.

18. What are some nutrient deficiencies associated with hypothyroidism?

Nutrient deficiencies associated with hypothyroidism include iodine, selenium, zinc, and vitamin D.

19. Can stress affect hypothyroidism?

Yes, stress can affect hypothyroidism by increasing cortisol levels, which can interfere with thyroid function.

20. What are some tips for meal planning with hypothyroidism?

Tips for meal planning with hypothyroidism include planning meals in advance, preparing meals in bulk, and consulting with a registered dietitian.

21. Can hypothyroidism affect digestion?

Yes, hypothyroidism can affect digestion by slowing down the digestive process.

22. What are some foods to avoid with Hashimoto's disease?

Individuals with Hashimoto's disease should avoid gluten, soy, and processed foods.

23. Can caffeine affect hypothyroidism?

Excessive caffeine intake can interfere with thyroid function, so it's important to consume caffeine in moderation.

24. What are some nutrient-dense snacks for individuals with hypothyroidism?

Nutrient-dense snacks for individuals with hypothyroidism include nuts, seeds, and fresh fruits and vegetables.

25. Can hypothyroidism affect fertility?

Yes, hypothyroidism can affect fertility by interfering with ovulation and menstrual cycles.

26. What are some nutrient-rich breakfast options for individuals with hypothyroidism?

Nutrient-rich breakfast options for individuals with hypothyroidism include eggs, smoothies, and oatmeal.

27. Can hypothyroidism cause hair loss?

Yes, hypothyroidism can cause hair loss due to a slowed metabolism.

28. What are some nutrient-rich lunch options for individuals with hypothyroidism?

Nutrient-rich lunch options for individuals with hypothyroidism include salads, soups, and sandwiches made with whole grain bread.

29. Can hypothyroidism cause fatigue?

Yes, hypothyroidism can cause fatigue due to a slowed metabolism.

30. What are some nutrient-rich dinner options for individuals with hypothyroidism?

Nutrient-rich dinner options for individuals with hypothyroidism include grilled fish, roasted vegetables, and quinoa bowls.

31. Can hypothyroidism cause depression?

Yes, hypothyroidism can cause depression due to a slowed metabolism and hormonal imbalances.

32. What are some nutrient-rich snack options for individuals with hypothyroidism?

Nutrient-rich snack options for individuals with hypothyroidism include hummus and vegetables, trail mix, and Greek yogurt.

33. Can hypothyroidism cause constipation?

Yes, hypothyroidism can cause constipation due to a slowed digestive process.

34. What are some nutrient-rich dessert options for individuals with hypothyroidism?

Nutrient-rich dessert options for individuals with hypothyroidism include fresh fruit, dark chocolate, and chia seed pudding.

35. Can hypothyroidism cause joint pain?

Yes, hypothyroidism can cause joint pain due to inflammation and hormonal imbalances.

36. What are some nutrient-rich smoothie options for individuals with hypothyroidism?

Nutrient-rich smoothie options for individuals with hypothyroidism include green smoothies made with spinach or kale, and smoothies made with berries and Greek yogurt.

37. Can hypothyroidism cause dry skin?

Yes, hypothyroidism can cause dry skin due to a slowed metabolism.

38. What are some nutrient-rich soup options for individuals with hypothyroidism?

Nutrient-rich soup options for individuals with hypothyroidism include vegetable soup, lentil soup, and chicken noodle soup made with whole grain noodles.

39. Can hypothyroidism cause brain fog?

Yes, hypothyroidism can cause brain fog due to hormonal imbalances and slowed metabolism.

40. What are some nutrient-rich snack options for individuals with hypothyroidism?

Nutrient-rich snack options for individuals with hypothyroidism include hard-boiled eggs, apple slices with almond butter, and roasted chickpeas.

Thank you immensely for choosing "Hypothyroidism Cookbook" as your guide toward healthier eating and well-being. Your support fuels my passion for creating resources that make a difference. Your reviews and feedback mean a lot; they not only assist others but also drive me to keep improving.

If you found this book beneficial, I kindly ask you to leave a review and recommend it to anyone else who might benefit from its insights. Your advocacy helps spread awareness and support to those in need. Thank you for being part of this incredible journey toward better health!

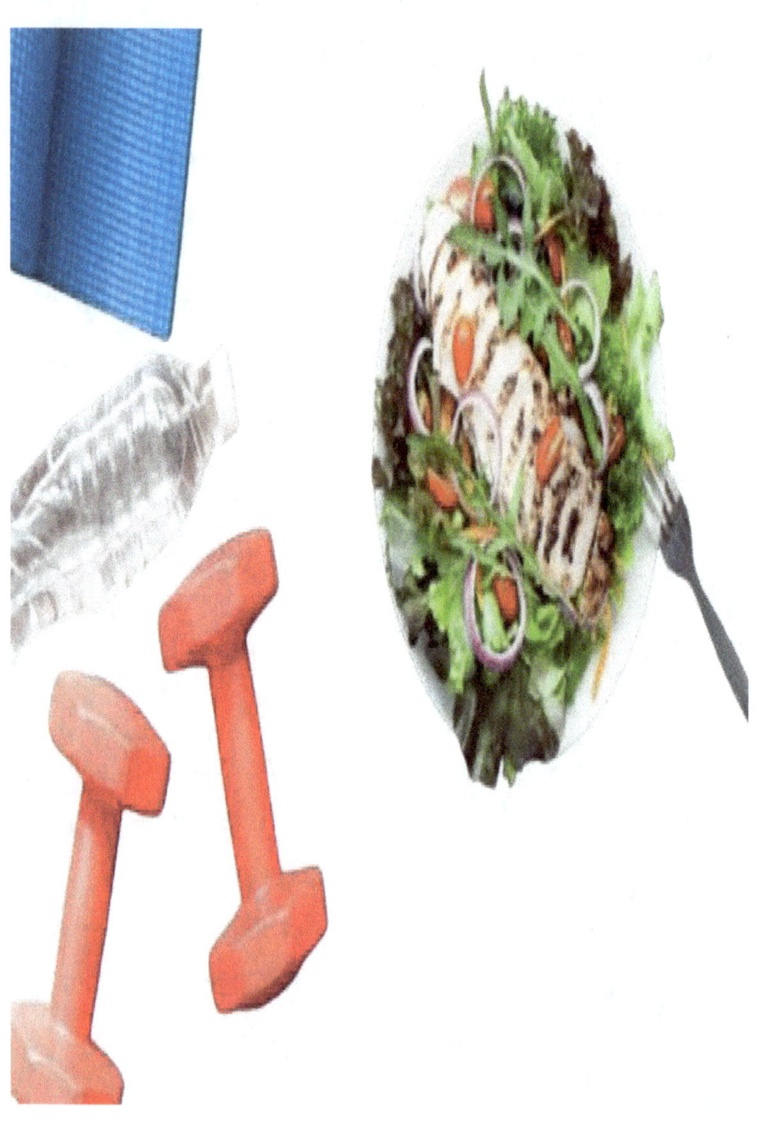